ALLERGIES AND INFECTIOUS DISEASES

CANDIDA *ALBICANS*

SYMPTOMS, CAUSES AND TREATMENT OPTIONS

Allergies and Infectious Diseases

Additional books in this series can be found on Nova's website under the Series tab.

Additional e-books in this series can be found on Nova's website under the e-book tab.

ALLERGIES AND INFECTIOUS DISEASES

CANDIDA *ALBICANS*

SYMPTOMS, CAUSES AND TREATMENT OPTIONS

LEON A. DIETRICH
AND
TIM S. FRIEDMANN
EDITORS

New York

For permission to use material from this book please contact us:
Telephone 631-231-7269; Fax 631-231-8175
Web Site: http://www.novapublishers.com

Additional color graphics may be available in the e-book version of this book.

Library of Congress Cataloging-in-Publication Data

ISBN: 978-1-62808-882-3

Library of Congress Control Number: 2013947024

Published by Nova Science Publishers, Inc. † New York

Contents

Preface

Infections due to the Candida species are the most common among fungal infections. Candida albicans is a yeast normally found as part of the skin microbiota, mouth, intestinal tract and vagina. Certain illnesses, stress, or medications can cause the out of control growth of Candida, producing infections that range from superficial to the systemic level, and potentially life-threatening diseases. In this book, the authors discuss the symptoms, causes and treatment options of Candida albincans including the role of Candida albicans biofilms in human disease; new developments in the pathogenesis of Candida albicans; a drug delivery approach for the treatment of Candida albicans; proteins and peptides as potential antifungals for treating Candida albicans infections; antifungal therapy of candidiasis with Amphotericin B; Candida albicans infection in the lower respiratory tract among HIV/AIDs patients in Nigeria; risk factors for vaginal candidiasis; symptomatology and therapy in candidiasis; microbial inactivation of the pathogen Candida albican in marine ecosystems; polyenes, azoles, and echinocandins for treating infections caused by Candida albicans and other Candida species; and new aspects of pathogenicity, interaction to antifungals, biofilms and preventive anti-Candida strategies.

Chapter I – In the human body, microbial cells outnumber human cells by a factor of ten. These human microbiome members include bacteria, archaea, and fungi. One of the major fungal members of the human microbiome is the yeast *Candida albicans. C. albicans* is a normal commensal member of the skin, gastrointestinal, oral, and female genitourinary tracts, and typically coexists on or within the human host without causing disease. However, changes in host immunity, environmental conditions, or alterations in other members of the host microbiota, can permit *C. albicans* to become pathogenic, causing diseases ranging from minor, superficial dermal and mucosal infections, to life-threatening systemic infections. *C. albicans* has traditionally been studied in the planktonic (or free-floating) state, however recent studies have revealed the importance of *C. albicans* growing in surface-associated communities, known as biofilms. *C. albicans* biofilms are intrinsically resistant to antifungal drugs, the host immune system, and other environmental stresses, making biofilm-based infections a significant challenge to treat in the clinic. *C. albicans* biofilms are a particularly serious problem for individuals with implanted medical devices, where the device serves as a substrate for biofilm growth. In this chapter, we describe how *C. albicans* has been studied *in vitro* and *in vivo*, review the literature on genetic regulation of *C. albicans* biofilm formation, and discuss the implications of polymicrobial biofilms that are made up of multiple *Candida* and/or bacterial species. We end this chapter by explaining the relevance of biofilms to human disease, describing interactions with the host immune system, and discussing current and promising future therapeutic options.

Chapter II – *Candida albicans* generally exists as a commensal organism and is present in approximately 50% of the human population. However, if host immunity is compromised, for example by AIDS, immunosuppressive drugs, or cancer chemotherapy, *C. albicans* can opportunistically cause recurrent candidiasis. In particular, the mortality rate from systemic candidiasis is very high due to a lack of effective diagnosis and treatment. Hence, there is an urgent need for clear elucidation of the virulence mechanisms of *C. albicans*.

Degradation of host tissues, evasion of the immune system, and dissemination via the blood stream are integral features of the overall virulence of *C. albicans*, and have been important areas of research. Among virulence factors of *C. albicans* that contribute to these processes, secreted aspartic proteases (Saps) are well-studied enzymes, and their roles have been evaluated in numerous investigations. Recent papers reveal unconventional properties of Saps and describe their roles in attacking host cells, degradation of host tissues, and immunity evasion. In addition to research concentrating on individual attributes, such as Saps, 'omics' approaches offer promising avenues to shed light on the complex virulence processes mentioned above. Analyses of overall virulence processes by omics technologies, for example proteomics, are beginning to uncover novel virulence attributes of *C. albicans*. This review describes new developments in the characterization of secreted aspartic proteases (Saps) and profiling of virulence processes by proteomics.

Chapter III – Infections due to *Candida* species are the most common among fungal infections. Although *Candida albicans* is a yeast normally found as part of the skin microbiota, mouth, intestinal tract and vagina. Certain illnesses, stress, or medications can cause the growth of *Candida* out of control producing infections that range from superficial to systemic level, and potentially life-threatening diseases. Not surprisingly, superficial candidiasis is a common reason for patient visits to dermatologists. On the other hand, the incidence of invasive *Candida* infections have continued to increase over the last decade within high risk patient groups, as those severely immunocompromised patients infected with HIV or under chemotherapy treatment, solid organ or haematopoietic stem cell transplant recipients, and patients in intensive care units. In this way early diagnosis and prompt initiation of antifungal therapy are essential factors to reduce morbidity and mortality. This chapter provides preliminary information on risk factor for *Candida* infections and symptoms. In addition, current knowledge about pharmaceutical formulation and drug delivery strategies on treatment of multiple forms of candidiasis is discussed.

Chapter IV – A multitude of peptides and proteins including lactoferrin, the lactoferrin-derived peptides lactoferrampin and lactoferricin and their chimera, and other lactoferrin-derived peptides; human, mammalian and submammalian defensins and cathelicidins , salivary histatin 5 and salivary glycoproteins, IQ-motif peptides, human thrombin C-terminal peptides, lysozyme, calprotectin, serum amyloid A, interleukin-2 and lipopolysaccharides have been found to be potential anti-Candida therapeutic agents.Their inhibitory actions on *Candida albicans* are reviewed.

Chapter V – Amphotericin B (AmB) remains the reference treatment for invasive fungal infections and the current guidelines for the treatment of haematogenous candidiasis recommend the use of AmB. Despite the diversity of antifungal drugs to cure these infections, only the action of AmB spectrum covers most of the *Candida* organisms, which are pathogenic species to humans. In addition, the cost of the treatment is an important element in the therapeutic strategy as fluconazole, voriconazole, and caspofungin are significantly more expensive than AmB. The conventional AmB-deoxycholate (Fungizone®) formulation which is a colloidal suspension of AmB has been available since 1958. While AmB is relatively cheaper, it has a large number of adverse effects, such as renal toxicity which constitutes the main reason for its restricted use. This toxicity is partially reduced with the antifungal lipid formulations. Unfortunately, their high cost (up to 90 times more expensive than Fungizone®) limits greatly their use in clinics and particularly in poor countries. To overcome this problem, some solutions have been proposed. However after exposure yeast cells to AmB, they were in a dormant state for 24 hours then the cells regrowth. Dormancy is one of the causes that reduce the effectiveness of the antifungal strategy. New formulation of amphotericin B based on the modulation of the physicochemical environment of the drug is discussed in this chapter in order to enhance the therapeutic index of amphotericin B.

Chapter VI – *Background: Candida albicans* is the the most pathogenic of about 68 species of *Candida.* It is a member of the normal flora of the skin, mucuos membranes, and gastrointestinal tract. *Candida* pneumonia is one of the most challenging of all the *Candida* infections. Primary *Candida* pneumonia refers to infections limited to the lungs, while secondary *Candida* pneumonia indicates lung involvement due to the movement of invasive *Candida* from other parts of the body.

Symptoms: The major clinical manifestations of primary *Candida* pneumonia are fever and tachypnoea. Radiologically, nonspecific patchy infiltrates can be seen. The only accepted criterion for the definitive diagnosis of *Candida* pneumonia is histological demonstration of the fungus in the lung.

Causes: Respiratory *Candida* infection can result from exogenous or endogenous source, hematogenous spread or by introduction of the pathogen into the lungs via catheters and lines.

Treatment options: Several factors must be considered when choosing antifungal agents for patients with HIV/AIDS. One important factor is efficacy. Antifungals are less efficacious in HIV-positive patients than in patients with cancer, and time for antifungal response is also more prolonged. In addition the relapse rate is higher in patients with HIV than in other patient's populations. Fluconazole is one of the most effective agents for the treatment of pulmonary candidiasis, especially in patients with AIDS. Fluconazole is active against most *Candida* species; however, resistant *C. albicans* strains have been isolated, primarily from AIDS patients under prolonged fluconazole treatment.

Aims and objectives: This study was designed to identify and characterize *Candida albicans* isolated from lower respiratory tract infections of HIV positive patients and to determine the prevalence rates of *Candida* infections among these subjects.

Materials and methods: Two early morning expectorate sputum samples were collected from 272 HIV positive subjects visiting the ART clinics and DOTS centre with cases of lower respiratory tract infection, over a period of 14 months from May, 2009 - July 2010 in Calabar. Subjects were recruited for this study upon approval by the Ethical Research Committee of the University of Calabar Teaching Hospital and obtaining written informed consent from the patients. Samples were processed by standard methods for isolation of *Candida*. Speciation was done by germ tube test, chlamydospore production on corn meal agar and sugar fermentation and assimilation tests using the Microexpress Candida identification kit (Tulip, India).

Results: Out of the 544 sputum samples collected from 272 subjects, *Candida* species were isolated from 40 (14.7%) and identified after confirming their growth in the second sample. The majority of *Candida* species among the *Candida* isolates were *Candida albicans* (80%) followed by *Candida tropicalis* 5(12.5%), *Candida dublinensis* 2(5.0%) and *Candida guilliermondii* 1(2.5%). The isolation rate of *Candida albicans* from sputum samples was found to be highest among subjects aged 25-34 years, followed by those aged 15-24 years. This study is the first of its kind to be carried out in Calabar and the South-South geopolitical region of Nigeria, and has shown that pulmonary albicans candidiasis is a health problem among HIV positive patients in Calabar.

Chapter VII – Vulvovaginal candidiasis is a leading cause of abnormal vaginal discharge. Inflammation of the vagina, as in any inflammatory sexually transmitted infection, increases the risk of acquisition of HIV. The study was set to establish the importance of the laboratory support in diagnosis of vaginal candidiasis in order to improve treatment of vaginal candidiasis in current syndromic management of abnormal vaginal discharge. A finding based on a prospective study of female genital swabs in some Primary Health Care Centers in Nigeria vis-à-vis a similar study in a University Teaching Hospital in Nigeria, December 2006 to December 2009 by the same author was made. Candida species were the most predominantly isolated organisms (60%) in the female genital discharges across the patients in both the primary health care centers and university teaching hospital in Nigeria. Also, young adults of age range 21 – 30 years and pregnant mothers constitute an important risk. Laboratory support was found to be necessary for a differential diagnosis or to confirm the clinical diagnosis of vaginal candidiasis. The finding shows that the high prevalence of vuvo-vaginal candidiasis cuts across social groups and necessitates a high index of diagnostic tools which is the laboratory.

Chapter VIII – The yeasts are represented by several genera, including *Candida* that presents various species causing infection in humans. However, some species colonize oral cavity, vaginal mucosa and gastrointestinal tract in healthy individuals. Particularly, *C. albicans* is considered the most frequent cause of superficial infections and life-threatening systemic infections. The clinical manifestations of oral candidiasis commonly are whitish plaques strongly or weakly adhered to the mucosa. The risk factors mainly include the wearing of dentures, extremes of age, prolonged antibiotic use, and underlying diseases specially *diabetes mellitus*. This infection may to evolve into oropharynx and the esophageal candidiasis. The vulvovaginal candidiasis clinically exhibits erythematous and pruriginous lesions, white discharge and unpleasant odor. The main predisposing factors for vulvovaginal candidiasis are use of antibiotics, oral contraception, pregnancy, hormone therapy and diseases as *diabetes mellitus*. However, neutropenia and damage of the gastrointestinal mucosa are considered conditions strictly related with the development of systemic (disseminated) candidiasis. Further risk factors include invasive medical device use, which allow direct access of the yeast to the bloodstream, broad-spectrum antibiotics, surgery trauma and even disrupts mucosal barriers. Diagnosis of invasive candidiasis and candidemia remains difficult and therefore prophylactic and pre-emptive therapies appear promising strategies in high-risk patients. Currently, treatment options to superficial and deep infections include antifungal agents from four licensed different classes: I) polyenes, represented for amphotericin B and several lipid formulations besides nystatin; II) azoles that include the imidazoles cetoconazole and miconazole, in addition to triazoles fluconazole, itraconazole and newer less toxic voriconazole, posaconazole and ravuconazole; III) echinocandins anidulafungin, caspofungin and micafungin and IV) the nucleoside analogue flucytosine that is only used as a part of a combination regimen. Due to the limited armory of the available antifungal and increasing reports of resistance, the choice of combination therapy has been explored to improve healing rates and allow reduction of the dose. Important considerations when choosing the antimycotic agents include the localization of the infection, the severity of disease, depletion of organ functions, previous exposure to antifungals, the identified fungal specie and your virulence factors, local resistance patterns and patient characteristics. We review the currently available data on pathogenesis, symptomatology and management strategies for superficial and invasive candidiasis and Candidemia.

Chapter IX – The saccharomycetes *Candida albicans* are widely distributed in marine ecosystems and their occurrence and distribution have been used as possible indicators of water pollution in the shoreline of aquatic ecosystems. Else, resistant forms of *Candida albicans* still well documented as a cause of skin infections both in human and animals and thought to be transmitted from contact with infested sands or sediments. Thus, there's actual vital interest in discovering new antimicrobial compounds with fewer environmental and toxicological risks and no resistance developped by the pathogens as *Candida albicans* and several marine natural products have been reported from large range of aquatic species with bioactivities in several species of pathogen fungi and bacteria. In present study we summarize actual data on diverse bio-activities against *Candida albicans* revealed in several species of marine algae, sponges, opistobranch mollusks and micro-epibionts.

Chapter X – Invasive fungal infection (IFI) is a serious problem since it is difficult to diagnose early and mortality is high. A variety of approaches are adopted for the therapy and management of IFI including prophylactic, empiric, preemptive, and directed strategies. Lipid formulations of amphotericin B (colloidal dispersion, lipid complex and liposomal) are better tolerated than amphotericin B deoxycholate and are equally effective. The lipid formulations have usually been used as second-line therapy in patients with refractory invasive candidiasis. Azole drugs are frequently used in cost-effective antifungal prophylaxis of patients with immunodeficiency and cancer that increase the susceptibility to invasive fungal infection. Fluconazole is the best known example. Echinocandins have desirable characteristics that render make them useful for treating Candida infections. Antibodies or their engineered derivatives directed against cell-wall polysaccharides and glycopeptides, and some protein epitopes of *Candida albicans* are seemingly a novel approach for prophylaxis against Candida infection and merit further in-depth studies.

Chapter XI – Own results, proposals, and conceptions published during last 5 years are summarized. *Candida albicans* and non-albicans Candida species isolated from urogenital tract of healthy people were compared in their interactions to antifungals (probiotic bacterial lectins [PBL] including bifidobacterial and lactobacillus lectins [BL, LL], phytolectins, antibiotics, lactobacilli) in suspensions and biofilms. Synergistic potential of antifungals against *Candida* species is presented. New prognostic and diagnostic features and criteria of *Candida albicans* strain pathogenicity according to both fungal behavior and fungal interaction to antimicrobials are proposed. Among *Candida* species strains tested, *C. albicans* strains reveal increased sensitivity to BL as well as to the block [ketokonazol, fluconazol] upon ranging antibiotic sensitivity.

Chapter XII – *Aims and Objectives:* The study was set to detect *Candida* species in female genital discharge and validate the associated risk factors by laboratory means .

Materials and Methods: A prospective study of female genital swabs collected from women with abnormal vaginal discharge (test group) and a control group who were attending gynecology, family planning, antenatal care or HIV/STI clinics of Aminu Kano Teaching

Hospital, Kano Nigeria and analysed for microscopy and culture in microbiology laboratory from December 2008 to December 2009. Data on epidemiologic indices were collected from the patients, using structured interviewer- administered questionnaires.

Results: Candida species were detected in the test group in 60% (n=600/1000) cases of infective vaginal discharge while 12% (120/1000) in the control group . The isolation rate of *Candida albicans* was 69% more than the non- albicans. Distribution of vaginal candidiasis in the test group, was prevalent in young adults age group of 21 to 30 years with 50% (n=300/600), in patients with pregnancy 38% (n=225/600) and patients with chronically debilitating illnesses 26% (n=157/600).

Conclusion: The result shows that vaginal candidiasis is quite common and *Candida albicans* is the most prevalent species. We therefore recommend early diagnosis and prompt treatment of vaginal candidiasis in all women clinics especially among the patients with chronic debilitating illness, pregnancy and young adults in order to avert the complications of vaginal candidiasis and reduce HIV transmission.

In: Candida *albicans*: Symptoms, Causes and Treatment Options ISBN: 978-1-62808-882-3
Editors: Leon A. Dietrich and Tim S. Friedmann

Chapter I

The Role of *Candida albicans* Biofilms in Human Disease

Emily P. Fox[1,2] and Clarissa J. Nobile[1*]

[1]Department of Microbiology and Immunology, University of California, San Francisco, San Francisco, CA, United States of America

[2]Tetrad Program, Department of Biochemistry and Biophysics, University of California, San Francisco, San Francisco, CA, United States of America

Abstract

In the human body, microbial cells outnumber human cells by a factor of ten. These human microbiome members include bacteria, archaea, and fungi. One of the major fungal members of the human microbiome is the yeast *Candida albicans*. *C. albicans* is a normal commensal member of the skin, gastrointestinal, oral, and female genitourinary tracts, and typically coexists on or within the human host without causing disease. However, changes in host immunity, environmental conditions, or alterations in other members of the host microbiota, can permit *C. albicans* to become pathogenic, causing diseases ranging from minor, superficial dermal and mucosal infections, to life-threatening systemic infections. *C. albicans* has traditionally been studied in the planktonic (or free-floating) state, however recent studies have revealed the importance of *C. albicans* growing in surface-associated communities, known as biofilms. *C. albicans* biofilms are intrinsically resistant to antifungal drugs, the host immune system, and other environmental stresses, making biofilm-based infections a significant challenge to treat in the clinic. *C. albicans* biofilms are a particularly serious problem for individuals with implanted medical devices, where the device serves as a substrate for biofilm growth. In this chapter, we describe how *C. albicans* has been studied *in vitro* and *in vivo*, review the literature on genetic regulation of *C. albicans* biofilm formation, and discuss the implications of polymicrobial biofilms that are made up of multiple *Candida* and/or bacterial species. We end this chapter by explaining the relevance of biofilms to

* Address correspondence to Clarissa J. Nobile (clarissa.nobile@ucsf.edu).

human disease, describing interactions with the host immune system, and discussing current and promising future therapeutic options.

1. Introduction

The word "biofilm" has garnered increasing recognition in the past decade as a descriptor of a common microbial state. In the broadest definition, a biofilm is a community of adherent cells with properties that are distinct from those of free-floating, or planktonic, cells [1].

In nature, biofilms are predominantly attached to a surface or found at liquid/air interfaces of bodies of water. In the clinic, biofilms of many microbial species have been associated with increased resistance to drugs and other stressors, compared to their planktonic counterparts [2, 3].

For decades, microbes were primarily studied in the planktonic state, but now it is recognized that most microbes naturally occur in the biofilm state [4]. These biofilms are found in diverse niches, including natural aquatic environments, manmade structures, and many of the tissues of plants and animals. The relationship between a biofilm community and its host is complex and may be beneficial, antagonistic, or both. Here we will focus on *Candida albicans* biofilms, which are notorious for colonizing implanted medical devices and seeding systemic infections in humans [5–8].

C. albicans is a normal member of the host microbiota, colonizing the oral cavity, skin, gastrointestinal tract, and female genitourinary tract [9–11]. In healthy individuals, *C. albicans* growth is generally innocuous, however, overgrowth due to changes in the host microbiota, local environment and the host immune response, can cause superficial dermal and mucosal infections, such as diaper rash, vaginal yeast infections, and thrush [12], [13]. In immunocompromised individuals, *C. albicans* can act as a life-threatening pathogen, invading the bloodstream and many of the major organs [7, 14].

Several groups have identified various genes that are required for normal biofilm formation in *C. albicans,* allowing us to better understand the genetic control of biofilms. Biofilms are resistant to most currently available antifungal drugs, and characterization of their genetic program provides an important avenue for identifying new therapeutic targets that are specific to the biofilm growth state. Here we will discuss how *C. albicans* biofilms develop, which genes contribute to biofilm formation, the role of biofilms in causing infection, and the current state of therapeutic treatment for biofilm-based infections.

2. Biofilm Formation *In Vitro* and *In Vivo*

Plastic catheters were first introduced in the 1940s [15], and in the 1980s the use of medically implanted devices such as catheters, heart valves, and joint replacements, constructed from polyurethane, polyethylene, and silicone, increased dramatically, along with the incidence of device-associated infections [15, 16]. Physicians noted that *C. albicans* growth on these devices was a significant medical problem that required removal and replacement of the infected device [17, 18]. It was only in the early 1990's that clinicians and scientists began to make the connection that the infection of these medical devices was the result of biofilm growth, and, at this time, no *in vitro* models existed to study this type of growth state in the laboratory. Then, in 1994, Hawser and Douglas published the first method for culturing a *C. albicans* biofilm *in vitro* [19]. In this assay, *C. albicans* cells are seeded on a silicone disc, submerged in media at 37°C, and allowed to adhere, statically, for one hour. Next, the unadhered cells are washed off and the adhered cells are allowed to develop into a biofilm over the course of one to three days. Later, *in vitro* biofilm models included shaking or flow of media to more closely mimic *in vivo* environments [20, 21]. *C. albicans* biofilms have been shown to grow on a vast array of substrates and in many different types of media *in vitro*, indicating that this organism is robust to forming biofilms under a wide range of environmental conditions [22–26]. Biofilm development *in vitro* follows a temporal progression [27, 28]. First, yeast cells adhere to the substrate, then, germ tubes form in response to temperature and cues in the media. As the cells divide, hyphal growth becomes more prominent and the mature biofilm becomes a mixture of yeast, pseudohyphae, and hyphae. As the biofilm matures, an extracellular matrix is secreted that coats the biofilm, protecting it from the environment [21]. Finally, dividing cells are released from the biofilm as dispersed cells, which then go on to seed new niches [29]. Figure 1 shows a confocal scanning laser microscopy (CSLM) side-view image of a mature *C. albicans* biofilm grown *in vitro*. Many different isolates of *C. albicans* and other *Candida* species have been successfully cultured *in vitro* under various environmental conditions [30, 31].

Models of *in vitro* biofilm formation have correlated reasonably well with biofilm formation *in vivo*. For example, *C. albicans* biofilms from denture stomatitis patients confirm the presence of yeast, hyphae and extracellular matrix in vivo [32]. Furthermore, biofilm architecture in two different animal catheter models (rat and rabbit) appears to include numerous yeast cells in the basal region, as well as hyphae and extracellular matrix extending throughout the biofilm [33, 34].

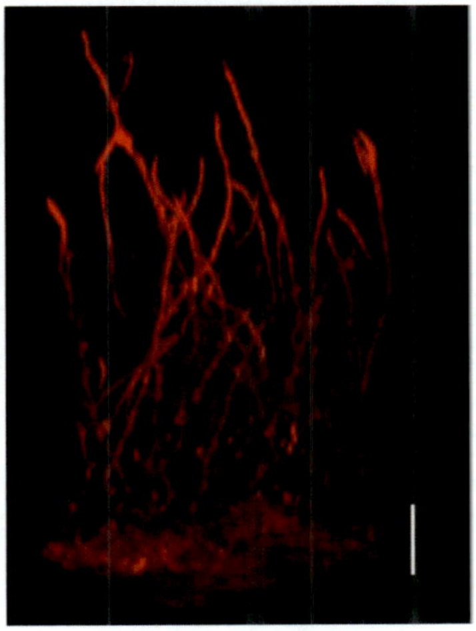

Figure 1. Morphology of a *C. albicans* biofilm in vitro. Wild-type *C. albicans* cells were seeded on bovine serum coated polystyrene in Brain Heart Infusion media supplemented with 5% Fetal Bovine Serum. Cells were adhered for 90 minutes, unadhered cells were washed off, and fresh media was added. Biofilms were allowed to develop, shaking, at 37°C, for 24 hours. Biofilms were stained with Concanavalin A - Alexa594 conjugate and imaged by Confocal Scanning Laser Microscopy. A z-stack image was assembled using Nikon NIS Elements software. Scale bar is 50 µm.

Currently, *in vivo* biofilm rodent models are most frequently used to validate *in vitro* results; these include central venous catheter models, denture models, oral mucosa models, subcutaneous models, vaginal models, and wound models [33, 35–39]. Overall, the basic components and the timing of biofilm development are similar *in vitro* and *in vivo*. Initial colonization *in vivo* occurs as yeast cells attach to a substrate, and within 24 - 72 hours the biofilm contains a mixture of yeast and hyphal cells, as well as extracellular matrix. Monoculture *Candida* biofilms may colonize formerly sterile sites, such as implanted medical devices. Biofilms formed on mucosal surfaces, however, are often polymicrobial and incorporate bacterial cells, as well as host cells and proteins [13, 36, 39–41].

3. Genetic Control of Biofilm Formation

Biofilms are complex communities of several different cell types with many properties that are distinct from those of planktonic cells, thus it is not surprising that the gene expression profile of biofilms is very different from that of planktonic cells. An overview of the genes involved in biofilm formation is shown in Table 1. Filamentous growth is essential for normal biofilm structure, thus it is not surprising that genes required for hyphal formation, such as *EFG1, TEC1,* and *HWP1*, are also important for biofilm formation [42–45]. Adhesion is another critical component of biofilm formation, and one transcriptional regulator of adhesins (Bcr1), and several downstream adhesins (Als1, Als3, and Hwp1) are required for normal biofilm development [28, 44, 46–48]. Twenty-nine additional transcriptional regulators have also been implicated in adherence, some of which are also important for mature biofilm development [49].

Biofilms are inherently resistant to antimicrobial agents and drugs. This is partly due to the upregulation of several genes associated with drug resistance, including the multidrug resistance (MDR) and *Candida* drug resistance (CDR) gene families, which encode multidrug efflux pumps [50].

Table 1.

Biofilm Process	**Genes**
Adhesion	*BCR1, ALS1, ALS3, HWP1, ACE2, ADA2, AHR1, ARG81, BRG1, CAS5, CRZ2, CZF1, DAL81, EFG1, FCR3, FGR27, GCN4, LEU3, MET4, NDT80, NOT3, NRG1, ROB1, SNF5, SUC1, TAF14, TEC1, TRY2, TRY3, TRY4, TRY5, TRY6, TYE7, UGA33, WAR1, ZAP1, ZCF28, ZCF31, ZCF34, ZCF39, ZCF8, ZFU2, ZNC1*
Filamentation	*EFG1, TEC1, NDT80, ROB1, HWP1*
Drug Resistance	*NDT80, MDR1, CDR1, CDR2, GSC1*
Matrix	*GSC1, BGL2, XOG1, PHR1, GCA1, GCA2, ZAP1*
Dispersion	*NRG1, UME6*
Transcriptional Regulation	*EFG1, TEC1, NDT80, BCR1, ROB1, BRG1, ACE2, ADA2, AHR1, ARG81, BCR1, BRG1, CAS5, CRZ2, CZF1, DAL81, EFG1, FCR3, FGR27, GCN4, LEU3, MET4, NDT80, NOT3, NRG1, ROB1, SNF5, SUC1, TAF14, TEC1, TRY2, TRY3, TRY4, TRY5, TRY6, TYE7, UGA33, WAR1, ZAP1, ZCF28, ZCF31, ZCF34, ZCF39, ZCF8, ZFU2, ZNC1*

Secreted extracellular matrix plays an additive role in drug resistance, acting as a direct physical barrier to drug penetration and contributing to the overall structural integrity of the biofilm [51–56].

One particular component of the *C. albicans* biofilm matrix, β-1,3-glucan, has been shown to play an important role in sequestering antifungal drugs. Genes involved in production and delivery of β-1,3-glucans include *FKS1/GSC1*, encoding a synthase, and *BGL2, XOG1*, and *PHR1*, encoding proteins involved in the transport and modification of β-glucans [57, 58]. There is currently one known transcriptional regulator of extracellular matrix production in *C. albicans*, Zap1, which is a negative regulator of biofilm matrix generation [59]. Zap1 likely controls aspects of extracellular matrix accumulation by regulating the glucoamylases, Gca1 and Gca2, which may directly contribute to the release of β-1,3-glucans into the matrix.

Cells are dispersed continuously throughout biofilm development, and are primarily thought to be in the yeast form [29]. While they are morphologically similar to suspension cultures of yeast cells, they appear to be phenotypically distinct from yeast cells. Dispersed cells are more adherent, form better biofilms, and are more virulent in a mouse model, compared to suspension cultures of yeast cells. Recently, the first two regulators of *C. albicans* biofilm dispersal were identified, Nrg1 and Ume6, where overexpression of either Nrg1 or Ume6 was able to increase the number of dispersed cells exiting the biofilm [29, 60].

In total, 40 transcriptional regulators have been described as playing some role in *Candida* biofilm function [61]. In 2012, Nobile et al. identified an interconnected network of six core transcriptional regulators (Efg1, Tec1, Bcr1, Ndt80, Brg1, and Rob1) that are essential for biofilm development [62]. Together, these six regulators directly bind to the promoters of ~1000 downstream target genes and indirectly regulate the expression of hundreds more. This work led to a major breakthrough in our understanding of how *Candida* biofilms are transcriptionally controlled. This network of genes encompasses those mentioned above, with roles in hyphal growth, adhesion, drug resistance and matrix production, but also includes newly identified target genes whose roles are yet to be worked out. Strikingly, the biofilm network target genes are significantly enriched for "young" genes (based on orthology mapping), suggesting that the ability of *C. albicans* to form biofilms evolved relatively rapidly in evolutionary timescales [62]. This may explain why *C. albicans* is one of only a few fungal species able to form biofilms within a mammalian host.

4. Polymicrobial Biofilms: Interactions between *C. Albicans* and Other Bacterial or Fungal Species

The major focus in studying *Candida* biofilms has been on *Candida albicans,* as it is the most commonly isolated species from the human host, accounting for 40-60% of *Candida* infections [63], [64]. However, several other *Candida* species are also capable of forming biofilms, and are also able to cause disease in humans. These include *Candida dubliniensis* and *Candida tropicalis*, which are the most closely related species to *C. albicans*, as well as *Candida parapsilosis, Candida guillermondii, Candida krusei,* and *Candida glabrata* [65–70]. Along with *C. albicans*, *C. parapsilosis* and *C. glabrata* are particularly prevalent in device-associated biofilm infections [8, 67]. Using culture conditions successful for *C.*

albicans, however, neither *C. parpsilosis* nor *C. glabrata* are capable of forming complex biofilms *in vitro* [19, 71]. Nevertheless, these species are able to form thick biofilms on implanted devices *in vivo* [72, 73]. *C. glabrata* and *C. kruseii*, in particular, are highly resistant to azole antifungal drugs, making treatment of biofilms containing these species exceedingly difficult. Over the last decade, non-*albicans* species have been increasingly isolated from numerous infection sites in the clinic, and the proportion of *C. albicans* to non-*albicans* species appears to vary by geographical location and human population [63, 74–77].

Candida species are able to form biofilms in monoculture in various, otherwise sterile *in vivo* locations, such as on implanted medical devices within a patient. However, many non-sterile sites of colonization, such as the oral cavity, intestinal mucosa, and vagina, are naturally inhabited by millions of bacterial, fungal and archaeal members of the microbiota, affording *Candida* many opportunities to interact with multiple microorganisms throughout these sites [78–82]. Likewise, numerous infections of typically sterile sites, such as wounds, medical devices, and internal organs, can also become polymicrobial, and *Candida* may encounter various species in these contexts as well [40, 41].

The best-characterized polymicrobial biofilms are found in the oral cavity, in the form of dental plaque, consisting of about a thousand bacterial species [83]. Polymicrobial oral biofilms are also associated with numerous infections of the oral cavity, including denture stomatitis, periodontitis, and dental caries [32], [84–88]. *C. albicans* is the predominant fungal species that is isolated from these oral infection sites, along with the numerous bacterial species. *C. albicans* has been studied pairwise *in vitro* with several commonly isolated oral bacteria, including *Streptococcus gordonii, Streptococcus mutans, Actinomyces viscosus,* and *Fusobacterium* species [89–93].

Outside of the oral cavity, *C. albicans* is also known to interact with many bacterial species found in the gut, such as *Enterococcus* and *Escherichia* species; those found in the vagina, such as *Lactobacillus* species; and those found in the lungs of cystic fibrosis patients, such as *Pseudomonas aeruginosa* [94–97]. Polymicrobial interactions observed *in vitro* include (1) direct cell-cell physical contact via adhesion, (2) alterations of the local environment through secretion of acids or nutritional metabolites that are stimulated by the presence of the other species, and (3) the secretion of signaling molecules that influence the behavior of the other species [98]. For example, *P. aeruginosa* physically binds to hyphal cells (but not yeast cells) of *C. albicans*, and is able to kill *C. albicans* hyphal cells by secreting phospholipase C and phenazine compounds [99]. In many polymicrobial examples, yeast-produced ethanol provides a carbon-source that enhances the growth of many bacterial species [100]. As mentioned above, secretion of small molecules is a common mode of inter-species and inter-kingdom communication, and several bacteria-specific molecules have been shown to inhibit hyphal formation in *C. albicans*. Some examples include homoserine lactones, made by gram-negative bacteria [101], trans-2-decenoic acid, made by *Streptococcus mutans* [102], and a currently unidentified secreted factor made by *Enterococcus faecalis* [95]. Farnesol, a sesquiterpene alcohol, which is made by *C. albicans* [103], is able to repress *C. albicans* biofilm formation and also has various effects on bacteria: it decreases production of pyocyanin, a virulence factor of *P. aeruginosa,* and it inhibits growth and biofilm formation of at least two *Staphylococcus* species [97, 104–107]. We have only just begun to discover the complex world of molecular communication between microbes. Better understanding of these interactions will increase our knowledge of microbial ecology and sociomicrobiology, and will lead to new and more pragmatic therapeutic approaches to combatting polymicrobial infections.

5. The Role of Biofilms in Infection

C. albicans is unusual in its ability to colonize diverse body sites with vastly different environmental conditions. These sites are diagrammed in Figure 2. It is unclear whether normal, non-pathogenic colonization of the oral, gastrointestinal, and vaginal tracts is associated with biofilm formation, but biofilms are certainly an important component of infectious overgrowth in many body sites. Biofilm-based infections in the host may be associated with either mucosal surfaces, such as the oral and vaginal cavities, or may be found on abiotic surfaces, such as implanted medical devices and prostheses. Oropharyngeal candidiasis (or thrush) is a common biofilm-based mucosal infection in immunocompromised individuals, and is found in ~90% of AIDS patients, ~5% of newborn babies, and ~10% of elderly patients [108, 109].

Vaginal yeast infections are composed of biofilms that adhere to the mucosa of the vaginal walls [39]. 75% of otherwise healthy adult women experience a vaginal yeast infection at least once in their lifetime, and 5 - 8% of adult women suffer from a recurrent form of yeast infection, known as recurrent vulvovaginal candidiasis [12, 110, 111].

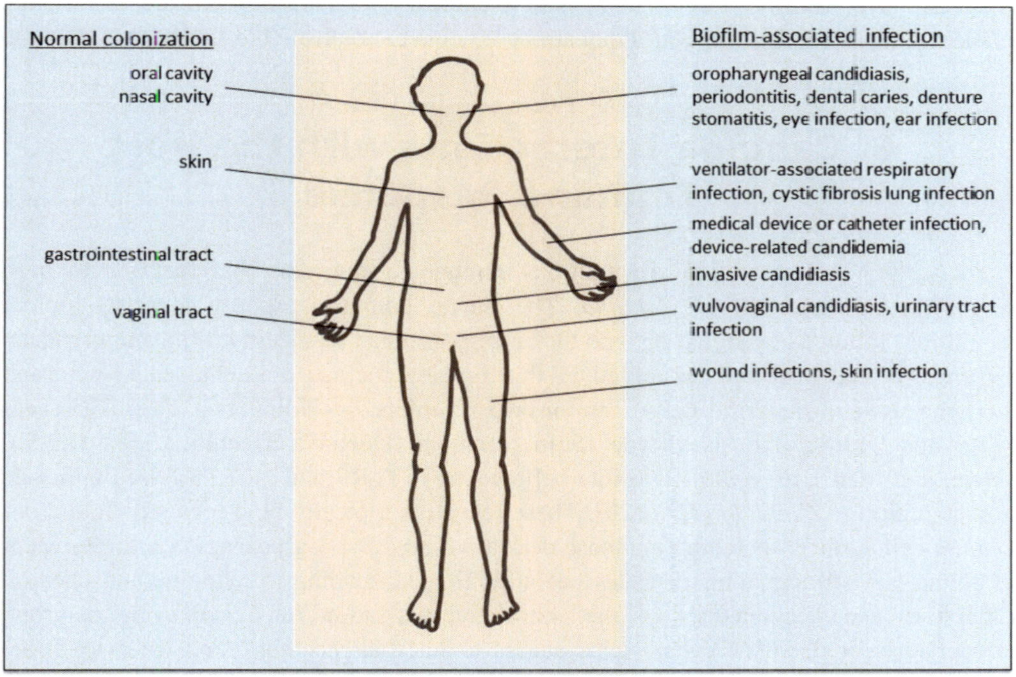

Figure 2. Sites of *Candida* biofilm growth in the human body. *Candida* biofilms are able to colonize diverse environments throughout the body. In healthy people, biofilms colonize exterior epithelial and mucosal surfaces. In immunocompromised people, *Candida* biofilms are capable of invading nearly every organ.

C. albicans also normally colonizes the entire intestinal tract, including the stomach, ileum, and cecum, and while it has not been determined whether this colonization is in the form of a mucosa-associated polymicrobial biofilm [9–11, 112], this is likely to be the case. Indeed, it is highly likely that the normal human microbiome exists predominantly in a structurally organized biofilm state, and that slight perturbations in the balance of species proportions may lead to disease states.

Biofilm growth on implanted medical devices is a particularly difficult infection to manage. Devices susceptible to *Candida* infection include heart valves, joint prostheses, dentures, contact lenses, and catheters of many kinds, including venous, urinary, and oral catheters [8, 67,72, 113–115]. *Candida* biofilms adhere tightly to these manmade surfaces, forming highly drug-resistant, adherent communities of cells. Dispersed cells from medical device-associated biofilms may travel into the bloodstream, causing candidemia, and in fact, at least half of all microbial bloodstream infections are associated with an indwelling medical device, and *Candida* species are the fourth most common cause of blood stream infections [65, 116, 117]. Device-associated candidemia is a serious medical problem, with estimated mortality rates between 19 and 50% [118–122]. Device-related, hospital-acquired (or nosocomial) infections with *Candida* are a particular problem in intensive care units (ICUs), affecting 15% of ICU patients [123]. Due to the inherently drug resistant nature of cells in biofilms, colonization of medical devices by *Candida* is extremely difficult to treat, and device removal and replacement is the current standard of care in most cases. Device removal is expensive and difficult for patients, especially in cases of surgically implanted devices [8], [115, 124, 125], and the development of new clinical care standards will depend on future advancements in novel therapeutics that are better able to eradicate biofilm-based infections.

6. *Candida* Interactions with the Host Immune Response

In healthy humans, there are multiple immune mechanisms that function to prevent overgrowth and invasion of *Candida.* The innate immune response involves molecular recognition, followed by signaling, and then a response that results in killing and/or clearance of *Candida.* The host cells involved in this process include epithelial cells, neutrophils, macrophages, and dendritic cells. Ten surface receptors, including two Toll-like receptors (TLR2 and TLR4), and six C-type lectin receptors (Dectin-1, Dectin-2, MR, DC-SIGN, Mincle, and MBL), as well as two internal receptors (TLR9 and NLRP3), are implicated in the recognition of *Candida* [126–129]. These receptors typically bind to sugars found on the *Candida* cell surface, including mannose derivatives and β-1,3-glucans. Once these receptors are bound, several signaling cascades become initiated, leading to cytokine and chemokine production, and phagocytosis of the yeast. Internalization of *Candida* by neutrophils, macrophages, or dendritic cells, yields access to internal receptors, and leads to TLR9 or NLRP3 inflammasome activation. These processes ultimately lead to the killing and clearance of *Candida* cells. While the innate immune response is a major player in fighting *Candida* infection, the adaptive response also plays an important role, and antibodies raised to extracellular proteins, such as mannan and aspartyl proteases, are critical in eliminating *Candida* and preventing its overgrowth [130].

The major biofilm infection of humans is mucosal candidiasis, and this type of infection largely activates the innate immune response, rather than the adaptive immune response. B-cell knockout mice, for example, are known to be resistant to mucosal candidiasis, yet susceptible to systemic infection [131]. In addition, in mucosal candidiasis, Th17 cells are required for the interleukin response, activating epithelial and mesenchymal cells to attract neturophils and secrete antimicrobial peptides [132]. Humans with mutations in genes encoding dectin-1 or Card9 (involved in sensing *Candida* and innate immune signaling) have decreased Th17 cell counts and increased susceptibility to mucocutaneous candidiasis [133], [134].

It is currently unknown how growth of *Candida* in the biofilm state affects interactions with the host immune system, but there are clues that indicate that aspects of biofilm formation may be protective against host defenses. Hyphal cells, for example, are an important component of biofilms, and they are able to penetrate epithelial cell layers during invasive growth [135, 136]. Hyphae are also able to mediate escape of the *Candida* cell from within phagocytic cells by physically piercing the phagocytic cell [137]. The gene *PRA1* and members of the secreted aspartyl protease (*SAP*) gene family are highly upregulated during biofilm formation, and are individually capable of blocking complement activation [138, 139]. *MSB2* is another highly upregulated gene in biofilms, encoding an adhesin-like protein involved in binding and blocking host-secreted antimicrobial peptides [140, 141]. Recently, it was shown that deletion of one of the major transcriptional regulators of biofilm development, Bcr1, caused *C. albicans* to be more susceptible to damage by leukocytes [142]. Although it is yet to be demonstrated that *Candida* biofilms interact differently with the immune system than planktonic cells, current transcriptional and phenotypic data support the idea that biofilms are geared to be more resistant to host immune factors, as biofilms have the ability to adhere tightly to surfaces, upregulate drug efflux pumps, and have altered metabolic properties [143].

Recent studies have begun to examine to what extent biofilm formation and virulence are linked. The National Institutes of Health has estimated that roughly 80% of human infections have a biofilm component (http://grants.nih.gov/grants/ guide/pa-files/PA-99-084.html). Biofilm formation is considered a virulence factor for mucosal infection, as adherence to the mucosal tissue is key [108, 144–146]. Bcr1, one of the transcriptional regulators required for biofilm formation, is also required for oral mucosal infection [142], and both Bcr1 and the biofilm regulator Efg1 are required for infection of the vaginal mucosa [39].

It is unclear whether biofilm formation is essential for colonization of the gut, but the evidence, thus far, suggests that the ability to form biofilms is not absolutely required for gut colonization, at least in the initial stages. A study performed in mice showed that the majority of cells initially colonizing the intestine appear to be in the yeast form [147], although whether these yeast-form cells further develop into biofilms over longer time periods is unknown. A more recent study showed that Efg1 and Tec1, two other transcriptional regulators required for biofilm formation, are not required for gut colonization of mice, and an *efg1* deletion mutant strain even over-proliferates compared to a reference strain in the gut [148, 149], suggesting that these two important biofilm regulators are not essential for gut colonization. However, another recent study showed that Cph2, a transcriptional regulator that is upregulated, but not required for biofilm growth *in vitro*, is important for efficient gut colonization [149]. Given the overlap between the targets of Efg1, Tec1, and Cph2, it is possible that Cph2 is the major biofilm regulator of the *in vivo* intestinal environment, and that Cph2 facilitates normal colonization and biofilm formation in the gut in the absence of the other two regulators.

While blood stream infections are not thought to be composed of biofilms, the majority of blood stream infections are associated with a biofilm infection of a medical device [8], [117, 150], so most blood stream infections are seeded from a biofilm somewhere else in the patient. Additionally, one study found that the ability to form biofilms was correlated with higher mortality in blood stream infections [65]. Overall, current evidence suggests that biofilms are an important virulence factor in *Candida* infections, but they are certainly not the only one. As we begin to understand more about biofilm formation *in vivo* and how *Candida* interacts with the host immune response, we will have a much more thorough understanding of how biofilms and virulence are linked *in vivo*.

7. Biofilm-Specific Therapeutics

There are currently four major classes of antifungal drugs used for treatment of *Candida* infections: azoles, polyenes, nucleoside analogs, and echinocandins [151–155]. Azoles, such as fluconazole, are fungistatic and block ergosterol synthesis by targeting the demethylase enzyme Erg11, which leads to an accumulation of toxic sterol pathway intermediates. Polyenes, such as Amphotericin B, are fungicidal and work by intercalating into membranes containing ergosterol, creating rigid pores that destroy the proton gradient, leading to leakage of the cytoplasm and other cell contents. Nucleoside analogs (or antimetabolites), such as 5-Flucytosine (5-FC), mimic nucleosides during nucleic acid synthesis. 5-FC specifically acts as a pyrimidine analog, disrupting fungal RNA, DNA, and protein synthesis, and ultimately leading to cell cycle arrest. 5-FC does not have intrinsic antifungal properties on its own, but becomes an antifungal when it is converted into 5-Fluorouracil (5-FU) inside fungal cells by a fungal cytosine deaminase. Echinocandins, such as Caspofungin, are the newest class of fungicidal drugs and work by targeting the synthesis of 1,3-β-D-glucan, an important component of the fungal cell wall.

Candida biofilms are up to 1000 times more resistant to antifungal drugs compared to planktonic cells [6], [155]. Thus far, echinocandins are the most effective drug class against *Candida* biofilms *in vitro*, and may be useful *in vivo* as well, although additional clinical studies are needed to assess their effectiveness against biofilms *in vivo* [156–158]. Current *in vivo* studies indicate that echinocandins are more effective than azoles or polyenes in reducing mortality due to invasive candidiasis, however removal of any biofilm-infected device appears to be the most important factor for improved patient outcome [159], suggesting that current antifungals are generally poor at eradicating *Candida* in the biofilm state. Indeed, current standard of care is to remove the medical device if a biofilm-based infection is suspected. As removal of medical devices is not always feasible, especially in cases where patients have surgically implanted devices, improving the treatment of biofilm-based infections will rely on the development of new drugs that are specifically effective against *Candida* biofilms.

Candida biofilm drug resistance is attributable to many distinguishing characteristics of biofilms. One fundamental characteristic is that biofilms express a genetic program unique to that of planktonic cells. Genes encoding several drug efflux pumps, including *MDR1, CDR1,* and *CDR2* are constitutively upregulated in biofilms. Several known drug target genes are also upregulated, including *ERG11* and *ERG25*, which are targets of the azole drugs [160]; as well as *KRE1* and *SKN1*, which are in the β-glucan synthesis pathway [161], and counteract the effects of polyenes. Fks1/Gsc1, which is involved in β-glucan production in the extracellular matrix, is also upregulated during biofilm formation; β-glucans in the matrix are able to sequester all four classes of antifungal drugs [53, 57]. Other than transcriptional changes in genes affecting drug pumps and drug targets, there are several other specific attributes of biofilms that contribute to drug resistance as well. First, the extracellular matrix is unique to biofilms and acts as a protective sheath that physically prevents drugs and other damaging agents from accessing the inner cells of the biofilm [21, 51], 52]. Second, biofilm cells enter a relatively sessile state in the mature stages of biofilm development, and this lowered metabolism creates an inherent resistance to drugs and damage [2], [162]. Finally, biofilms generate a subpopulation of dormant and highly resistant cells, known as "persister cells," which are thought to survive biofilm disruption and are then able to go on to seed new niches for biofilm growth [163, 164].

Recent work has sought to develop vaccines against *Candida* infection. Thus far, the GPI-anchored adhesin, Als3, appears to be a promising vaccine target. Als3 is important for *Candida* adherence to manmade surfaces and endothelial and epithelial cells; and deletion of *ALS3* results in decreased biofilm formation [46, 165].

Vaccination with recombinant Als3-N has been effective at protecting mice from mucosal candidiasis as well as disseminated infection [166], and has successfully passed through a Phase I human trial. Another vaccine target currently under investigation is the secreted aspartyl protease, Sap2. Vaccination with recombinant, truncated rSap2t has successfully protected rats against vulvovaginal candidiasis [167]. Phase I human trials are currently underway for this Sap2-based vaccine. If development of a vaccine against *Candida* is successful, vaccination of at risk patient populations may be a powerful tool for prevention of biofilm-related infections.

Current standard of care for treating *Candida* biofilm infections varies depending on the site of infection, the age and health of the patient, and the species of *Candida* [168]. An azole-based antifungal is standard treatment for non-neutropenic adults, and echinocandins are reserved for neutropenic patients, those with azole-resistant infections, and those infected with *Candida glabrata*, which is generally azole-resistant [169–171]. Amphotericin B or fluconazole are generally used to treat neonatal candidiasis, however the use of echinocandins is also on the rise in neonatal intensive care units [170, 172]. Fluconazole is recommended prophylactically for transplant recipients and those entering the intensive care units [170, 173].

Candidiasis of implanted medical devices may require treatment of the device (such as in antifungal lock therapy of catheters), administration of azole or echinocandin drugs, and possible removal and replacement of the device [8, 67, 114, 124, 174]. The advances in development of new antifungal drugs and therapeutic protocols have successfully reduced mortality and morbidity for *Candida*-related infections to some degree. However, ongoing work in new drug discovery and vaccine development is key to outpacing emerging drug resistance seen in multiple *Candida* species [154], [175], and for developing therapeutics that are effective against *Candida* biofilms.

Acknowledgments

We are grateful for the availability of the Nikon Imaging Center (NIC) at UCSF, where the confocal scanning laser microscopy images were taken. This study was supported by NIH grants T32AI060537, K99AI100896 and R01AI083311.

References

[1] D. López, H. Vlamakis, and R. Kolter, "Biofilms.," *Cold Spring Harbor perspectives in biology*, vol. 2, no. 7, p. a000398, Jul. 2010.

[2] J. W. Costerton, P. S. Stewart, and E. P. Greenberg, "Bacterial biofilms: a common cause of persistent infections.," *Science (New York, N.Y.)*, vol. 284, no. 5418, pp. 1318–22, May 1999.

[3] R. Wolcott, J. W. Costerton, D. Raoult, and S. J. Cutler, "The polymicrobial nature of biofilm infection," pp. 1–6, 2012.

[4] R. Kolter and E. P. Greenberg, "Microbial sciences: the superficial life of microbes.," *Nature*, vol. 441, no. 7091, pp. 300–2, May 2006.

[5] J. C. O. Sardi, L. Scorzoni, T. Bernardi, a M. Fusco-Almeida, and M. J. S. Mendes Giannini, "Candida species: current epidemiology, pathogenicity, biofilm formation, natural antifungal products and new therapeutic options.," *Journal of medical microbiology*, vol. 62, no. Pt 1, pp. 10–24, Jan. 2013.

[6] S. Tobudic, C. Kratzer, A. Lassnigg, and E. Presterl, "Antifungal susceptibility of Candida albicans in biofilms.," *Mycoses*, vol. 55, no. 3, pp. 199–204, May 2012.

[7] J. Kim and P. Sudbery, "Candida albicans, a major human fungal pathogen.," *Journal of microbiology (Seoul, Korea)*, vol. 49, no. 2, pp. 171–7, Apr. 2011.

[8] R. Cauda, "Candidaemia in patients with an inserted medical device.," *Drugs*, vol. 69 Suppl 1, pp. 33–8, Jan. 2009.

[9] M. E. Bertholf and M. J. Stafford, "Colonization of Candida albicans in vagina, rectum, and mouth.," *The Journal of family practice*, vol. 16, no. 5, pp. 919–24, May 1983.

[10] M. Zwolinska-Wcisło, A. Budak, J. Bogdał, D. Trojanowska, and J. Stachura, "Fungal colonization of gastric mucosa and its clinical relevance.," *Medical science monitor : international medical journal of experimental and clinical research*, vol. 7, no. 5, pp. 982–8.

[11] M. J. Kennedy and P. a Volz, "Ecology of Candida albicans gut colonization: inhibition of Candida adhesion, colonization, and dissemination from the gastrointestinal tract by bacterial antagonism.," *Infection and immunity*, vol. 49, no. 3, pp. 654–63, Sep. 1985.

[12] J. D. Sobel, S. Faro, R. W. Force, B. Foxman, W. J. Ledger, P. R. Nyirjesy, B. D. Reed, and P. R. Summers, "Vulvovaginal candidiasis " Epidemiologic , diagnostic, and therapeutic considerations," vol. 178, no. 2, pp. 203–211, 1998.

[13] J. A. Vazquez and J. D. Sobel, "*Mucosal candidiasis*," vol. 16, pp. 793–820, 2002.

[14] S. K. Fridkin and W. R. Jarvis, "Epidemiology of nosocomial fungal infections.," *Clinical microbiology reviews*, vol. 9, no. 4, pp. 499–511, Oct. 1996.

[15] T. S. Elliott, "Intravascular-device infections.," *Journal of medical microbiology*, vol. 27, no. 3, pp. 161–7, Nov. 1988.

[16] D. a Goldmann and G. B. Pier, "Pathogenesis of infections related to intravascular catheterization.," *Clinical Microbiology Reviews*, vol. 6, no. 2, pp. 176–192, 1993.

[17] N. S. Tchekmedyian, K. Newman, M. R. Moody, J. W. Costerton, J. Aisner, S. C. Schimpff, and W. P. Reed, "Special studies of the Hickman catheter of a patient with recurrent bacteremia and candidemia.," *The American journal of the medical sciences*, vol. 291, no. 6, pp. 419–24, Jun. 1986.

[18] G. Reid, J. D. Denstedt, Y. S. Kang, D. Lam, and C. Nause, "Microbial adhesion and biofilm formation on ureteral stents in vitro and in vivo.," *The Journal of urology*, vol. 148, no. 5, pp. 1592–4, Nov. 1992.

[19] S. P. Hawser and L. J. Douglas, "Biofilm formation by Candida species on the surface of catheter materials in vitro.," *Infection and immunity*, vol. 62, no. 3, pp. 915–21, Mar. 1994.

[20] H. Bernhardt, K. Zimmermann, and M. Knoke, "The continuous flow culture as an in vitro model in experimental mycology.," *Mycoses*, vol. 42 Suppl 2, pp. 29–32, Jan. 1999.

[21] S. P. Hawser, G. S. Baillie, and L. J. Douglas, "Production of extracellular matrix by Candida albicans biofilms.," *Journal of Medical Microbiology*, vol. 47, no. 3, pp. 253–256, 1998.

[22] H. D. Rose, "Venous catheter-associated candidemia.," *The American journal of the medical sciences*, vol. 275, no. 3, pp. 265–9.

[23] B. H. Sen, K. E. Safavi, and L. S. Spångberg, "Colonization of Candida albicans on cleaned human dental hard tissues.," *Archives of oral biology*, vol. 42, no. 7, pp. 513–20, Jul. 1997.

[24] H. J. Busscher, G. I. Geertsema-Doornbusch, and H. C. van der Mei, "Adhesion to silicone rubber of yeasts and bacteria isolated from voice prostheses: influence of salivary conditioning films.," *Journal of biomedical materials research*, vol. 34, no. 2, pp. 201–9, Feb. 1997.

[25] H. Nikawa, T. Yamamoto, T. Hamada, M. B. Rahardjo, and H. Murata, "Commercial denture cleansers--cleansing efficacy against Candida albicans biofilm and compatibility wit soft denture-lining materials.," *The International journal of prosthodontics*, vol. 8, no. 5, pp. 434–44.

[26] L. A. Wilson, A. D. Sawant, and D. G. Ahearn, "Comparative efficacies of soft contact lens disinfectant solutions against microbial films in lens cases.," *Archives of ophthalmology*, vol. 109, no. 8, pp. 1155–7, Aug. 1991.

[27] G. S. Baillie and L. J. Douglas, "Role of dimorphism in the development of Candida albicans biofilms.," *Journal of Medical Microbiology*, vol. 48, no. 7, pp. 671–9, 1999.

[28] J. Chandra, D. M. Kuhn, P. K. Mukherjee, L. L. Hoyer, T. McCormick, and M. a Ghannoum, "Biofilm formation by the fungal pathogen Candida albicans: development, architecture, and drug resistance.," *Journal of bacteriology*, vol. 183, no. 18, pp. 5385–94, Sep. 2001.

[29] P. Uppuluri, A. K. Chaturvedi, A. Srinivasan, M. Banerjee, A. K. Ramasubramaniam, J. R. Köhler, D. Kadosh, and J. L. Lopez-Ribot, "Dispersion as an important step in the Candida albicans biofilm developmental cycle.," *PLoS pathogens*, vol. 6, no. 3, p. e1000828, Mar. 2010.

[30] G. Ramage, E. Mowat, B. Jones, C. Williams, and J. Lopez-Ribot, "Our current understanding of fungal biofilms.," *Critical reviews in microbiology*, vol. 35, no. 4, pp. 340–55, Jan. 2009.

[31] M. a El-Azizi, S. E. Starks, and N. Khardori, "Interactions of Candida albicans with other Candida spp. and bacteria in the biofilms.," *Journal of applied microbiology*, vol. 96, no. 5, pp. 1067–73, Jan. 2004.

[32] G. Ramage, K. Tomsett, B. L. Wickes, J. L. López-Ribot, and S. W. Redding, "Denture stomatitis: a role for Candida biofilms," *Oral Surgery, Oral Medicine, Oral Pathology, Oral Radiology, and Endodontology*, vol. 98, no. 1, pp. 53–59, Jul. 2004.

[33] D. Andes, J. Nett, P. Oschel, R. Albrecht, K. Marchillo, and A. Pitula, "Development and characterization of an in vivo central venous catheter Candida albicans biofilm model.," *Infection and immunity*, vol. 72, no. 10, pp. 6023–31, Oct. 2004.

[34] M. K. Schinabeck, L. A. Long, M. A. Hossain, J. Chandra, P. K. Mukherjee, S. Mohamed, and M. A. Ghannoum, "Rabbit model of Candida albicans biofilm infection: liposomal amphotericin B antifungal lock therapy.," *Antimicrobial agents and chemotherapy*, vol. 48, no. 5, pp. 1727–32, May 2004.

[35] J. E. Nett, K. Marchillo, C. a Spiegel, and D. R. Andes, "Development and validation of an in vivo Candida albicans biofilm denture model.," *Infection and immunity*, vol. 78, no. 9, pp. 3650–9, Sep. 2010.

[36] A. Dongari-Bagtzoglou, H. Kashleva, P. Dwivedi, P. Diaz, and J. Vasilakos, "Characterization of mucosal Candida albicans biofilms.," *PloS one*, vol. 4, no. 11, p. e7967, Jan. 2009.

[37] J. Chandra, L. Long, M. A. Ghannoum, and P. K. Mukherjee, "A rabbit model for evaluation of catheter-associated fungal biofilms.," *Virulence*, vol. 2, no. 5, pp. 466–74, 2011.

[38] M. Ricicová, S. Kucharíková, H. Tournu, J. Hendrix, H. Bujdáková, J. Van Eldere, K. Lagrou, and P. Van Dijck, "Candida albicans biofilm formation in a new in vivo rat model.," *Microbiology (Reading, England)*, vol. 156, no. Pt 3, pp. 909–19, Mar. 2010.

[39] M. M. Harriott, E. a Lilly, T. E. Rodriguez, P. L. Fidel, and M. C. Noverr, "Candida albicans forms biofilms on the vaginal mucosa.," *Microbiology (Reading, England)*, vol. 156, no. Pt 12, pp. 3635–44, Dec. 2010.

[40] B. M. Peters, M. A. Jabra-Rizk, G. a O'May, J. W. Costerton, and M. E. Shirtliff, "Polymicrobial interactions: impact on pathogenesis and human disease.," *Clinical microbiology reviews*, vol. 25, no. 1, pp. 193–213, Jan. 2012.

[41] M. M. Harriott and M. C. Noverr, "Importance of Candida-bacterial polymicrobial biofilms in disease.," *Trends in microbiology*, vol. 19, no. 11, pp. 557–63, Nov. 2011.

[42] G. Ramage, K. VandeWalle, J. L. López-Ribot, and B. L. Wickes, "The filamentation pathway controlled by the Efg1 regulator protein is required for normal biofilm formation and development in Candida albicans.," *FEMS microbiology letters*, vol. 214, no. 1, pp. 95–100, Aug. 2002.

[43] A. Schweizer, S. Rupp, B. N. Taylor, M. Röllinghoff, and K. Schröppel, "The TEA/ATTS transcription factor CaTec1p regulates hyphal development and virulence in Candida albicans.," *Molecular microbiology*, vol. 38, no. 3, pp. 435–45, Nov. 2000.

[44] C. J. Nobile, J. E. Nett, D. R. Andes, and A. P. Mitchell, "Function of Candida albicans adhesin Hwp1 in biofilm formation.," *Eukaryotic cell*, vol. 5, no. 10, pp. 1604–10, Oct. 2006.

[45] C. J. Nobile and A. P. Mitchell, "Regulation of cell-surface genes and biofilm formation by the C. albicans transcription factor Bcr1p.," *Current biology : CB*, vol. 15, no. 12, pp. 1150–5, Jun. 2005.

[46] C. J. Nobile, D. R. Andes, J. E. Nett, F. J. Smith, F. Yue, Q.-T. Phan, J. E. Edwards, S. G. Filler, and A. P. Mitchell, "Critical role of Bcr1-dependent adhesins in C. albicans biofilm formation in vitro and in vivo.," *PLoS pathogens*, vol. 2, no. 7, p. e63, Jul. 2006.

[47] C. J. Nobile, H. a Schneider, J. E. Nett, D. C. Sheppard, S. G. Filler, D. R. Andes, and A. P. Mitchell, "Complementary adhesin function in C. albicans biofilm formation.," *Current biology : CB*, vol. 18, no. 14, pp. 1017–24, Jul. 2008.

[48] X. Zhao, K. J. Daniels, S. Oh, C. B. Green, K. M. Yeater, D. R. Soll, and L. L. Hoyer, "Candida albicans Als3p is required for wild-type biofilm formation on silicone elastomer surfaces.," *Microbiology (Reading, England)*, vol. 152, no. Pt 8, pp. 2287–99, Aug. 2006.

[49] J. S. Finkel, W. Xu, D. Huang, E. M. Hill, J. V Desai, C. a Woolford, J. E. Nett, H. Taff, C. T. Norice, D. R. Andes, F. Lanni, and A. P. Mitchell, "Portrait of Candida albicans adherence regulators.," *PLoS pathogens*, vol. 8, no. 2, p. e1002525, Feb. 2012.

[50] G. Ramage, "Investigation of multidrug efflux pumps in relation to fluconazole resistance in Candida albicans biofilms," *Journal of Antimicrobial Chemotherapy*, vol. 49, no. 6, pp. 973–980, Jun. 2002.

[51] G. S. Baillie and L. J. Douglas, "Matrix polymers of Candida biofilms and their possible role in biofilm resistance to antifungal agents.," *The Journal of antimicrobial chemotherapy*, vol. 46, no. 3, pp. 397–403, Sep. 2000.

[52] M. A. Al-Fattani and L. J. Douglas, "Biofilm matrix of Candida albicans and Candida tropicalis: chemical composition and role in drug resistance.," *Journal of medical microbiology*, vol. 55, no. Pt 8, pp. 999–1008, Aug. 2006.

[53] J. Nett, L. Lincoln, K. Marchillo, R. Massey, K. Holoyda, B. Hoff, M. VanHandel, and D. Andes, "Putative role of beta-1,3 glucans in Candida albicans biofilm resistance.," *Antimicrobial agents and chemotherapy*, vol. 51, no. 2, pp. 510–20, Feb. 2007.

[54] J. E. Nett, H. Sanchez, M. T. Cain, and D. R. Andes, "Genetic basis of Candida biofilm resistance due to drug-sequestering matrix glucan.," *The Journal of infectious diseases*, vol. 202, no. 1, pp. 171–5, Jul. 2010.

[55] K. F. Mitchell, H. T. Taff, M. a Cuevas, E. L. Reinicke, H. Sanchez, and D. R. Andes, "Role of matrix β-1,3 glucan in antifungal resistance of non-albicans Candida biofilms.," *Antimicrobial agents and chemotherapy*, vol. 57, no. 4, pp. 1918–20, Apr. 2013.

[56] C. J. Nobile and A. P. Mitchell, "Microbial biofilms: e pluribus unum.," *Current biology: CB*, vol. 17, no. 10, pp. R349–53, May 2007.

[57] J. E. Nett, K. Crawford, K. Marchillo, and D. R. Andes, "Role of Fks1p and matrix glucan in Candida albicans biofilm resistance to an echinocandin, pyrimidine, and polyene.," *Antimicrobial agents and chemotherapy*, vol. 54, no. 8, pp. 3505–8, Aug. 2010.

[58] H. T. Taff, J. E. Nett, R. Zarnowski, K. M. Ross, H. Sanchez, M. T. Cain, J. Hamaker, A. P. Mitchell, and D. R. Andes, "A Candida biofilm-induced pathway for matrix glucan delivery: implications for drug resistance.," *PLoS pathogens*, vol. 8, no. 8, p. e1002848, Jan. 2012.

[59] C. J. Nobile, J. E. Nett, A. D. Hernday, O. R. Homann, J.-S. Deneault, A. Nantel, D. R. Andes, A. D. Johnson, and A. P. Mitchell, "Biofilm matrix regulation by Candida albicans Zap1.," *PLoS biology*, vol. 7, no. 6, p. e1000133, Jun. 2009.

[60] P. Uppuluri, C. G. Pierce, D. P. Thomas, S. S. Bubeck, S. P. Saville, and J. L. Lopez-Ribot, "The transcriptional regulator Nrg1p controls Candida albicans biofilm formation and dispersion.," *Eukaryotic cell*, vol. 9, no. 10, pp. 1531–7, Oct. 2010.

[61] E. P. Fox and C. J. Nobile, "A sticky situation: Untangling the transcriptional network controlling biofilm development in Candida albicans.," *Transcription*, vol. 3, no. 6, pp. 1–8, Nov. 2012.

[62] C. J. Nobile, E. P. Fox, J. E. Nett, T. R. Sorrells, Q. M. Mitrovich, A. D. Hernday, B. B. Tuch, D. R. Andes, and A. D. Johnson, "A Recently Evolved Transcriptional Network Controls Biofilm Development in Candida albicans," *Cell*, vol. 148, no. 1–2, pp. 126–138, 2012.

[63] M. Pfaller, D. Neofytos, D. Diekema, N. Azie, H.-U. Meier-Kriesche, S.-P. Quan, and D. Horn, "Epidemiology and outcomes of candidemia in 3648 patients: data from the Prospective Antifungal Therapy (PATH Alliance®) registry, 2004-2008.," *Diagnostic microbiology and infectious disease*, vol. 74, no. 4, pp. 323–31, Dec. 2012.

[64] A. S. Chitnis, S. S. Magill, J. R. Edwards, T. M. Chiller, S. K. Fridkin, and F. C. Lessa, "Trends in Candida central line-associated bloodstream infections among NICUs, 1999-2009.," *Pediatrics*, vol. 130, no. 1, pp. e46–52, Jul. 2012.

[65] M. Tumbarello, B. Posteraro, E. M. Trecarichi, B. Fiori, M. Rossi, R. Porta, K. de Gaetano Donati, M. La Sorda, T. Spanu, G. Fadda, R. Cauda, and M. Sanguinetti, "Biofilm production by Candida species and inadequate antifungal therapy as predictors of mortality for patients with candidemia.," *Journal of clinical microbiology*, vol. 45, no. 6, pp. 1843–50, Jun. 2007.

[66] J. Perlroth, B. Choi, and B. Spellberg, "Nosocomial fungal infections: epidemiology, diagnosis, and treatment.," *Medical mycology: official publication of the International Society for Human and Animal Mycology*, vol. 45, no. 4, pp. 321–46, Jun. 2007.

[67] E. M. Kojic, R. O. Darouiche, and C. Biofilms, "Candida Infections of Medical Devices," *Society*, vol. 17, no. 2, pp. 255–267, 2004.

[68] L. Masala, R. Luzzati, L. Maccacaro, L. Antozzi, E. Concia, and R. Fontana, "Nosocomial cluster of Candida guillermondii fungemia in surgical patients.," *European journal of clinical microbiology & infectious diseases: official publication of the European Society of Clinical Microbiology*, vol. 22, no. 11, pp. 686–8, Nov. 2003.

[69] M. A. Jabra-Rizk, W. A. Falkler, W. G. Merz, A. A. Baqui, J. I. Kelley, and T. F. Meiller, "Retrospective identification and characterization of Candida dubliniensis isolates among Candida albicans clinical laboratory isolates from human immunodeficiency virus (HIV)-infected and non-HIV-infected individuals.," *Journal of clinical microbiology*, vol. 38, no. 6, pp. 2423–6, Jun. 2000.

[70] D. C. Coleman, D. J. Sullivan, D. E. Bennett, G. P. Moran, H. J. Barry, and D. B. Shanley, "Candidiasis: the emergence of a novel species, Candida dubliniensis.," *AIDS (London, England)*, vol. 11, no. 5, pp. 557–67, Apr. 1997.

[71] L. C. F. Paiva, P. G. Vidigal, L. Donatti, T. I. E. Svidzinski, and M. E. L. Consolaro, "Assessment of in vitro biofilm formation by Candida species isolates from vulvovaginal candidiasis and ultrastructural characteristics.," *Micron (Oxford, England: 1993)*, vol. 43, no. 2–3, pp. 497–502, Feb. 2012.

[72] S. M. L. Seddiki, Z. Boucherit-Otmani, K. Boucherit, S. Badsi-Amir, M. Taleb, and D. Kunkel, "Assessment of the types of catheter infectivity caused by Candida species and their biofilm formation. First study in an intensive care unit in Algeria.," *International journal of general medicine*, vol. 6, pp. 1–7, Jan. 2013.

[73] A. H. Paulitsch, B. Willinger, B. Zsalatz, E. Stabentheiner, E. Marth, and W. Buzina, "In-vivo Candida biofilms in scanning electron microscopy.," *Medical mycology: official publication of the International Society for Human and Animal Mycology*, vol. 47, no. 7, pp. 690–6, Nov. 2009.

[74] M. E. Falagas, N. Roussos, and K. Z. Vardakas, "Relative frequency of albicans and the various non-albicans Candida spp among candidemia isolates from inpatients in various parts of the world: a systematic review.," *International journal of infectious diseases: IJID: official publication of the International Society for Infectious Diseases*, vol. 14, no. 11, pp. e954–66, Nov. 2010.

[75] M. T. Montagna, G. Caggiano, G. Lovero, O. De Giglio, C. Coretti, T. Cuna, R. Iatta, M. Giglio, L. Dalfino, F. Bruno, and F. Puntillo, "Epidemiology of invasive fungal infections in the intensive care unit: results of a multicenter Italian survey (AURORA Project).," *Infection*, vol. 41, no. 3, pp. 645–53, Jun. 2013.

[76] F. Guo, Y. Yang, Y. Kang, B. Zang, W. Cui, B. Qin, Y. Qin, Q. Fang, T. Qin, D. Jiang, W. Li, Q. Gu, H. Zhao, D. Liu, X. Guan, J. Li, X. Ma, K. Yu, D. Chan, J. Yan, Y. Tang, W. Liu, R. Li, and H. Qiu, "Invasive candidiasis in intensive care units in China: a multicentre prospective observational study.," *The Journal of antimicrobial chemotherapy*, Mar. 2013.

[77] M. Nucci, F. Queiroz-Telles, T. Alvarado-Matute, I. N. Tiraboschi, J. Cortes, J. Zurita, M. Guzman-Blanco, M. E. Santolaya, L. Thompson, J. Sifuentes-Osornio, J. I. Echevarria, and A. L. Colombo, "Epidemiology of candidemia in Latin America: a laboratory-based survey.," *PloS one*, vol. 8, no. 3, p. e59373, Jan. 2013.

[78] J. C. Stearns, M. D. J. Lynch, D. B. Senadheera, H. C. Tenenbaum, M. B. Goldberg, D. G. Cvitkovitch, K. Croitoru, G. Moreno-Hagelsieb, and J. D. Neufeld, "Bacterial biogeography of the human digestive tract.," *Scientific reports*, vol. 1, p. 170, Jan. 2011.

[79] M. a Ghannoum, R. J. Jurevic, P. K. Mukherjee, F. Cui, M. Sikaroodi, A. Naqvi, and P. M. Gillevet, "Characterization of the oral fungal microbiome (mycobiome) in healthy individuals.," *PLoS pathogens*, vol. 6, no. 1, p. e1000713, Jan. 2010.

[80] G. B. Huffnagle and M. C. Noverr, "The emerging world of the fungal microbiome.," *Trends in microbiology*, May 2013.

[81] R. F. Lamont, J. D. Sobel, R. a Akins, S. S. Hassan, T. Chaiworapongsa, J. P. Kusanovic, and R. Romero, "The vaginal microbiome: new information about genital tract flora using molecular based techniques.," *BJOG: an international journal of obstetrics and gynaecology*, vol. 118, no. 5, pp. 533–49, Apr. 2011.

[82] S. R. Gill, M. Pop, R. T. Deboy, P. B. Eckburg, P. J. Turnbaugh, B. S. Samuel, J. I. Gordon, D. a Relman, C. M. Fraser-Liggett, and K. E. Nelson, "Metagenomic analysis of the human distal gut microbiome.," *Science (New York, N.Y.)*, vol. 312, no. 5778, pp. 1355–9, Jun. 2006.

[83] C. J. Seneviratne, C. F. Zhang, and L. P. Samaranayake, "Dental plaque biofilm in oral health and disease.," *The Chinese journal of dental research: the official journal of the*

Scientific Section of the Chinese Stomatological Association (CSA), vol. 14, no. 2, pp. 87–94, Jan. 2011.

[84] T. Pereira-Cenci, D. M. Deng, E. A. Kraneveld, E. M. M. Manders, A. A. Del Bel Cury, J. M. Ten Cate, and W. Crielaard, "The effect of Streptococcus mutans and Candida glabrata on Candida albicans biofilms formed on different surfaces.," *Archives of oral biology*, vol. 53, no. 8, pp. 755–64, Aug. 2008.

[85] L. Coulthwaite and J. Verran, "Potential pathogenic aspects of denture plaque," *British Journal of Biomedical Science*, vol. 64, no. 4, pp. 180–189, 2007.

[86] H. Lamfon, Z. Al-Karaawi, M. McCullough, S. R. Porter, and J. Pratten, "Composition of in vitro denture plaque biofilms and susceptibility to antifungals.," *FEMS microbiology letters*, vol. 242, no. 2, pp. 345–51, Jan. 2005.

[87] H. Senpuku, a. Sogame, E. Inoshita, Y. Tsuha, H. Miyazaki, and N. Hanada, "Systemic Diseases in Association with Microbial Species in Oral Biofilm from Elderly Requiring Care," *Gerontology*, vol. 49, no. 5, pp. 301–309, 2003.

[88] S. Offenbacher, "Periodontal diseases: pathogenesis.," *Annals of periodontology / the American Academy of Periodontology*, vol. 1, no. 1, pp. 821–78, Nov. 1996.

[89] L. M. Jarosz, D. M. Deng, H. C. van der Mei, W. Crielaard, and B. P. Krom, "Streptococcus mutans competence-stimulating peptide inhibits Candida albicans hypha formation.," *Eukaryotic cell*, vol. 8, no. 11, pp. 1658–64, Nov. 2009.

[90] C. V Bamford, A. d'Mello, A. H. Nobbs, L. C. Dutton, M. M. Vickerman, and H. F. Jenkinson, "Streptococcus gordonii modulates Candida albicans biofilm formation through intergeneric communication.," *Infection and immunity*, vol. 77, no. 9, pp. 3696–704, Sep. 2009.

[91] S. K. Filoche, K. J. Soma, and C. H. Sissons, "Caries-related plaque microcosm biofilms developed in microplates.," *Oral microbiology and immunology*, vol. 22, no. 2, pp. 73–9, Apr. 2007.

[92] Z. M. Thein, Y. H. Samaranayake, and L. P. Samaranayake, "Effect of oral bacteria on growth and survival of Candida albicans biofilms.," *Archives of oral biology*, vol. 51, no. 8, pp. 672–80, Aug. 2006.

[93] N. J. Grimaudo and W. E. Nesbitt, "Coaggregation of Candida albicans with oral Fusobacterium species.," *Oral microbiology and immunology*, vol. 12, no. 3, pp. 168–73, Jun. 1997.

[94] H. M. H. N. Bandara, J. Y. Y. Yau, R. M. Watt, L. J. Jin, and L. P. Samaranayake, "Escherichia coli and its lipopolysaccharide modulate in vitro Candida biofilm formation.," *Journal of medical microbiology*, vol. 58, no. Pt 12, pp. 1623–31, Dec. 2009.

[95] M. R. Cruz, C. E. Graham, B. C. Gagliano, M. C. Lorenz, and D. a Garsin, "Enterococcus faecalis inhibits hyphal morphogenesis and virulence of Candida albicans.," *Infection and immunity*, vol. 81, no. 1, pp. 189–200, Jan. 2013.

[96] M. E. Falagas, G. I. Betsi, and S. Athanasiou, "Probiotics for prevention of recurrent vulvovaginal candidiasis: a review.," *The Journal of antimicrobial chemotherapy*, vol. 58, no. 2, pp. 266–72, Aug. 2006.

[97] G. McAlester, F. O'Gara, and J. P. Morrissey, "Signal-mediated interactions between Pseudomonas aeruginosa and Candida albicans.," *Journal of medical microbiology*, vol. 57, no. Pt 5, pp. 563–9, May 2008.

[98] A. Y. Peleg, D. a Hogan, and E. Mylonakis, "Medically important bacterial-fungal interactions.," *Nature reviews. Microbiology*, vol. 8, no. 5, pp. 340–9, May 2010.

[99] D. a Hogan and R. Kolter, "Pseudomonas-Candida interactions: an ecological role for virulence factors.," *Science (New York, N.Y.)*, vol. 296, no. 5576, pp. 2229–32, Jun. 2002.

[100] M. G. Smith, S. G. Des Etages, and M. Snyder, "Microbial synergy via an ethanol-triggered pathway.," *Molecular and cellular biology*, vol. 24, no. 9, pp. 3874–84, May 2004.

[101] D. a Hogan, A. Vik, and R. Kolter, "A Pseudomonas aeruginosa quorum-sensing molecule influences Candida albicans morphology.," *Molecular microbiology*, vol. 54, no. 5, pp. 1212–23, Dec. 2004.

[102] R. Vílchez, A. Lemme, B. Ballhausen, V. Thiel, S. Schulz, R. Jansen, H. Sztajer, and I. Wagner-Döbler, "Streptococcus mutans inhibits Candida albicans hyphal formation by the fatty acid signaling molecule trans-2-decenoic acid (SDSF).," *Chembiochem: a European journal of chemical biology*, vol. 11, no. 11, pp. 1552–62, Jul. 2010.

[103] G. Ramage, S. P. Saville, B. L. Wickes, J. L. López-ribot, and L. Lo, "Inhibition of Candida albicans Biofilm Formation by Farnesol, a Quorum-Sensing Molecule Inhibition of Candida albicans Biofilm Formation by Farnesol, a Quorum-Sensing Molecule," 2002.

[104] C. Cugini, D. K. Morales, and D. a Hogan, "Candida albicans-produced farnesol stimulates Pseudomonas quinolone signal production in LasR-defective Pseudomonas aeruginosa strains.," *Microbiology (Reading, England)*, vol. 156, no. Pt 10, pp. 3096–107, Oct. 2010.

[105] M. A. Jabra-Rizk, T. F. Meiller, C. E. James, and M. E. Shirtliff, "Effect of farnesol on Staphylococcus aureus biofilm formation and antimicrobial susceptibility.," *Antimicrobial agents and chemotherapy*, vol. 50, no. 4, pp. 1463–9, Apr. 2006.

[106] C. Cugini, M. W. Calfee, J. M. Farrow, D. K. Morales, E. C. Pesci, and D. a Hogan, "Farnesol, a common sesquiterpene, inhibits PQS production in Pseudomonas aeruginosa.," *Molecular microbiology*, vol. 65, no. 4, pp. 896–906, Aug. 2007.

[107] F. I. a Gomes, P. Teixeira, J. Azeredo, and R. Oliveira, "Effect of farnesol on planktonic and biofilm cells of Staphylococcus epidermidis.," *Current microbiology*, vol. 59, no. 2, pp. 118–22, Aug. 2009.

[108] S. Ganguly and A. P. Mitchell, "Mucosal biofilms of Candida albicans.," *Current opinion in microbiology*, vol. 14, no. 4, pp. 380–5, Aug. 2011.

[109] L. P. Samaranayake, W. K. Leung, and L. Jin, "Oral mucosal fungal infections," vol. 49, pp. 39–59, 2009.

[110] J. D. Sobel, "Pathogenesis of Recurrent Vulvovaginal Candidiasis.," *Current infectious disease reports*, vol. 4, no. 6, pp. 514–519, Dec. 2002.

[111] J. D. Sobel, "Vulvovaginal candidosis.," *Lancet*, vol. 369, no. 9577, pp. 1961–71, Jun. 2007.

[112] H. Bernhardt and M. Knoke, "Mycological aspects of gastrointestinal microflora.," *Scandinavian journal of gastroenterology. Supplement*, vol. 222, pp. 102–6, Jan. 1997.

[113] D. C. Burton, J. R. Edwards, A. Srinivasan, S. K. Fridkin, and C. V Gould, "Trends in catheter-associated urinary tract infections in adult intensive care units-United States, 1990-2007.," *Infection control and hospital epidemiology: the official journal of the Society of Hospital Epidemiologists of America*, vol. 32, no. 8, pp. 748–56, Aug. 2011.

[114] S. Shoham, "Invasive Candidiasis in Patients with Implants," *Current Fungal Infection Reports*, vol. 5, no. 1, pp. 12–17, Nov. 2010.

[115] I. Raad, H. Hanna, and D. Maki, "Intravascular catheter-related infections: advances in diagnosis, prevention , and management," 2007.

[116] M. A. Pfaller, D. J. Diekema, R. N. Jones, H. S. Sader, A. C. Fluit, and R. J. Hollis, "International Surveillance of Bloodstream Infections Due to Candida Species : Frequency of Occurrence and In Vitro Susceptibilities to Fluconazole , Ravuconazole , and Voriconazole of Isolates Collected from 1997 through 1999 in the SENTRY Antimicrobial S," vol. 39, no. 9, pp. 3254–3259, 2001.

[117] M. J. Richards, J. R. Edwards, D. H. Culver, and R. P. Gaynes, "Nosocomial infections in combined medical-surgical intensive care units in the United States.," *Infection control and hospital epidemiology: the official journal of the Society of Hospital Epidemiologists of America*, vol. 21, no. 8, pp. 510–5, Aug. 2000.

[118] J. Morgan, M. I. Meltzer, B. D. Plikaytis, A. N. Sofair, S. Huie-White, S. Wilcox, L. H. Harrison, E. C. Seaberg, R. A. Hajjeh, and S. M. Teutsch, "Excess mortality, hospital stay, and cost due to candidemia: a case-control study using data from population-based candidemia surveillance.," *Infection control and hospital epidemiology: the official journal of the Society of Hospital Epidemiologists of America*, vol. 26, no. 6, pp. 540–7, Jun. 2005.

[119] R. a Hajjeh, A. N. Sofair, L. H. Harrison, G. M. Lyon, B. a Arthington-Skaggs, S. a Mirza, M. Phelan, J. Morgan, W. Lee-Yang, M. a Ciblak, L. E. Benjamin, L. Thomson Sanza, S. Huie, S. F. Yeo, M. E. Brandt, and D. W. Warnock, "Incidence of Bloodstream Infections Due to Candida Species and In Vitro Susceptibilities of Isolates Collected from 1998 to 2000 in a Population-Based Active Surveillance Program," *Journal of Clinical Microbiology*, vol. 42, no. 4, pp. 1519–1527, 2004.

[120] O. Gudlaugsson, S. Gillespie, K. Lee, J. Vande Berg, J. Hu, S. Messer, L. Herwaldt, M. Pfaller, and D. Diekema, "Attributable mortality of nosocomial candidemia, revisited.," *Clinical infectious diseases: an official publication of the Infectious Diseases Society of America*, vol. 37, no. 9, pp. 1172–7, Nov. 2003.

[121] D. Pittet and R. P. Wenzel, "Nosocomial bloodstream infections. Secular trends in rates, mortality, and contribution to total hospital deaths.," *Archives of internal medicine*, vol. 155, no. 11, pp. 1177–84, Jun. 1995.

[122] S. B. Wey, M. Mori, M. A. Pfaller, R. F. Woolson, and R. P. Wenzel, "Hospital-Acquired Candidemia The Attributable," vol. 52242, 1988.

[123] O. Eloy, S. Marque, B. Mourvilliers, P. Pina, P. Y. Allouch, B. Pangon, J. P. Bedos, and J. C. Ghnassia, "Contribution of the Pittet's index, antigen assay, IgM, and total antibodies in the diagnosis of invasive candidiasis in intensive care unit," *Journal de Mycologie Médicale / Journal of Medical Mycology*, vol. 16, no. 3, pp. 113–118, Sep. 2006.

[124] L. a Mermel, M. Allon, E. Bouza, D. E. Craven, P. Flynn, N. P. O'Grady, I. I. Raad, B. J. a Rijnders, R. J. Sherertz, and D. K. Warren, "Clinical practice guidelines for the diagnosis and management of intravascular catheter-related infection: 2009 Update by the Infectious Diseases Society of America.," *Clinical infectious diseases: an official publication of the Infectious Diseases Society of America*, vol. 49, no. 1, pp. 1–45, Jul. 2009.

[125] T. J. Walsh and J. H. Rex, "All catheter-related candidemia is not the same: assessment of the balance between the risks and benefits of removal of vascular catheters.," *Clinical infectious diseases: an official publication of the Infectious Diseases Society of America*, vol. 34, no. 5, pp. 600–2, Mar. 2002.

[126] S.-C. Cheng, L. a B. Joosten, B.-J. Kullberg, and M. G. Netea, "Interplay between Candida albicans and the mammalian innate host defense.," *Infection and immunity*, vol. 80, no. 4, pp. 1304–13, Apr. 2012.

[127] M. G. Netea and L. Maródi, "Innate immune mechanisms for recognition and uptake of Candida species.," *Trends in immunology*, vol. 31, no. 9, pp. 346–53, Sep. 2010.

[128] S. G. Filler, "Candida-host cell receptor-ligand interactions.," *Current opinion in microbiology*, vol. 9, no. 4, pp. 333–9, Aug. 2006.

[129] N. A. R. Gow, F. L. van de Veerdonk, A. J. P. Brown, and M. G. Netea, "Candida albicans morphogenesis and host defence: discriminating invasion from colonization.," *Nature reviews. Microbiology*, vol. 10, no. 2, pp. 112–22, Feb. 2012.

[130] A. Casadevall, M. Feldmesser, and L. Pirofski, "Induced humoral immunity and vaccination against major human fungal pathogens.," *Current opinion in microbiology*, vol. 5, no. 4, pp. 386–91, Aug. 2002.

[131] R. D. Wagner, a Vazquez-Torres, J. Jones-Carson, T. Warner, and E. Balish, "B cell knockout mice are resistant to mucosal and systemic candidiasis of endogenous origin but susceptible to experimental systemic candidiasis.," *The Journal of infectious diseases*, vol. 174, no. 3, pp. 589–97, Sep. 1996.

[132] N. Hernández-Santos and S. L. Gaffen, "Th17 cells in immunity to Candida albicans.," *Cell host & microbe*, vol. 11, no. 5, pp. 425–35, May 2012.

[133] B. Ferwerda, G. Ferwerda, T. S. Plantinga, J. A. Willment, A. B. van Spriel, H. Venselaar, C. C. Elbers, M. D. Johnson, A. Cambi, C. Huysamen, L. Jacobs, T. Jansen, K. Verheijen, L. Masthoff, S. A. Morré, G. Vriend, D. L. Williams, J. R. Perfect, L. A. B. Joosten, C. Wijmenga, J. W. M. van der Meer, G. J. Adema, B. J. Kullberg, G. D. Brown, and M. G. Netea, "Human dectin-1 deficiency and mucocutaneous fungal infections.," *The New England journal of medicine*, vol. 361, no. 18, pp. 1760–7, Oct. 2009.

[134] E.-O. Glocker, A. Hennigs, M. Nabavi, A. A. Schäffer, C. Woellner, U. Salzer, D. Pfeifer, H. Veelken, K. Warnatz, F. Tahami, S. Jamal, A. Manguiat, N. Rezaei, A. A. Amirzargar, A. Plebani, N. Hannesschläger, O. Gross, J. Ruland, and B. Grimbacher, "A homozygous CARD9 mutation in a family with susceptibility to fungal infections.," *The New England journal of medicine*, vol. 361, no. 18, pp. 1727–35, Oct. 2009.

[135] Q. T. Phan, R. a Fratti, N. V Prasadarao, J. E. Edwards, and S. G. Filler, "N-cadherin mediates endocytosis of Candida albicans by endothelial cells.," *The Journal of biological chemistry*, vol. 280, no. 11, pp. 10455–61, Mar. 2005.

[136] S. G. Filler and D. C. Sheppard, "Fungal invasion of normally non-phagocytic host cells.," *PLoS pathogens*, vol. 2, no. 12, p. e129, Dec. 2006.

[137] S. Ghosh, D. H. M. L. P. Navarathna, D. D. Roberts, J. T. Cooper, A. L. Atkin, T. M. Petro, and K. W. Nickerson, "Arginine-induced germ tube formation in Candida albicans is essential for escape from murine macrophage line RAW 264.7.," *Infection and immunity*, vol. 77, no. 4, pp. 1596–605, Apr. 2009.

[138] S. Luo, A. Hartmann, H.-M. Dahse, C. Skerka, and P. F. Zipfel, "Secreted pH-regulated antigen 1 of Candida albicans blocks activation and conversion of complement C3.,"

Journal of immunology (Baltimore, Md. : 1950), vol. 185, no. 4, pp. 2164–73, Aug. 2010.

[139] K. Gropp, L. Schild, S. Schindler, B. Hube, P. F. Zipfel, and C. Skerka, "The yeast Candida albicans evades human complement attack by secretion of aspartic proteases.," *Molecular immunology*, vol. 47, no. 2–3, pp. 465–75, Dec. 2009.

[140] M. Swidergall, A. M. Ernst, and J. F. Ernst, "Candida albicans mucin Msb2 is a broad-range protectant against antimicrobial peptides.," *Antimicrobial agents and chemotherapy*, vol. 49, no. June, Jun. 2013.

[141] E. Szafranski-Schneider, M. Swidergall, F. Cottier, D. Tielker, E. Román, J. Pla, and J. F. Ernst, "Msb2 shedding protects Candida albicans against antimicrobial peptides.," *PLoS pathogens*, vol. 8, no. 2, p. e1002501, Feb. 2012.

[142] P. Dwivedi, A. Thompson, Z. Xie, H. Kashleva, S. Ganguly, A. P. Mitchell, and A. Dongari-Bagtzoglou, "Role of Bcr1-activated genes Hwp1 and Hyr1 in Candida albicans oral mucosal biofilms and neutrophil evasion.," *PloS one*, vol. 6, no. 1, p. e16218, Jan. 2011.

[143] F. L. Mayer, D. Wilson, and B. Hube, "Candida albicans pathogenicity mechanisms.," *Virulence*, vol. 4, no. 2, pp. 119–28, Feb. 2013.

[144] F. Hasan, I. Xess, X. Wang, N. Jain, and B. C. Fries, "Biofilm formation in clinical Candida isolates and its association with virulence.," *Microbes and infection / Institut Pasteur*, vol. 11, no. 8–9, pp. 753–61, 2009.

[145] M. M. Harriott and M. C. Noverr, "Ability of Candida albicans mutants to induce Staphylococcus aureus vancomycin resistance during polymicrobial biofilm formation.," *Antimicrobial agents and chemotherapy*, vol. 54, no. 9, pp. 3746–55, Sep. 2010.

[146] J. W. M. van der Meer, F. L. van de Veerdonk, L. a B. Joosten, B.-J. Kullberg, and M. G. Netea, "Severe Candida spp. infections: new insights into natural immunity.," *International journal of antimicrobial agents*, vol. 36 Suppl 2, pp. S58–62, Dec. 2010.

[147] S. J. White, A. Rosenbach, P. Lephart, D. Nguyen, A. Benjamin, S. Tzipori, M. Whiteway, J. Mecsas, and C. a Kumamoto, "Self-regulation of Candida albicans population size during GI colonization.," *PLoS pathogens*, vol. 3, no. 12, p. e184, Dec. 2007.

[148] J. V Pierce, D. Dignard, M. Whiteway, and C. a Kumamoto, "Normal adaptation of Candida albicans to the murine gastrointestinal tract requires Efg1p-dependent regulation of metabolic and host defense genes.," *Eukaryotic cell*, vol. 12, no. 1, pp. 37–49, Jan. 2013.

[149] A. Rosenbach, D. Dignard, J. V Pierce, M. Whiteway, and C. a Kumamoto, "Adaptations of Candida albicans for growth in the mammalian intestinal tract.," *Eukaryotic cell*, vol. 9, no. 7, pp. 1075–86, Jul. 2010.

[150] J. J. Picazo, F. González-Romo, and F. J. Candel, "Candidemia in the critically ill patient.," *International journal of antimicrobial agents*, vol. 32 Suppl 2, pp. S83–5, Nov. 2008.

[151] M. A. Jabra-Rizk, W. A. Falkler, and T. F. Meiller, "Fungal biofilms and drug resistance.," *Emerging infectious diseases*, vol. 10, no. 1, pp. 14–9, Jan. 2004.

[152] T. C. White, K. a Marr, and R. a Bowden, "Clinical, cellular, and molecular factors that contribute to antifungal drug resistance.," *Clinical microbiology reviews*, vol. 11, no. 2, pp. 382–402, Apr. 1998.

[153] S. C.-A. Chen, M. A. Slavin, and T. C. Sorrell, "Echinocandin antifungal drugs in fungal infections: a comparison.," *Drugs*, vol. 71, no. 1, pp. 11–41, Jan. 2011.

[154] L. E. Cowen, "The evolution of fungal drug resistance: modulating the trajectory from genotype to phenotype.," *Nature reviews. Microbiology*, vol. 6, no. 3, pp. 187–98, Mar. 2008.

[155] G. Ramage, R. Rajendran, L. Sherry, and C. Williams, "Fungal biofilm resistance.," *International journal of microbiology*, vol. 2012, p. 528521, Jan. 2012.

[156] S. P. Bachmann, K. VandeWalle, G. Ramage, T. F. Patterson, B. L. Wickes, J. R. Graybill, and J. L. López-Ribot, "In vitro activity of caspofungin against Candida albicans biofilms.," *Antimicrobial agents and chemotherapy*, vol. 46, no. 11, pp. 3591–6, Nov. 2002.

[157] P. Uppuluri, A. K. Chaturvedi, and J. L. Lopez-Ribot, "Design of a simple model of Candida albicans biofilms formed under conditions of flow: development, architecture, and drug resistance.," *Mycopathologia*, vol. 168, no. 3, pp. 101–9, Sep. 2009.

[158] S. Kucharíková, N. Sharma, I. Spriet, J. Maertens, P. Van Dijck, and K. Lagrou, "Activities of systemically administered echinocandins against in vivo mature Candida albicans biofilms developed in a rat subcutaneous model.," *Antimicrobial agents and chemotherapy*, vol. 57, no. 5, pp. 2365–8, May 2013.

[159] D. R. Andes, N. Safdar, J. W. Baddley, G. Playford, A. C. Reboli, J. H. Rex, J. D. Sobel, P. G. Pappas, and B. J. Kullberg, "Impact of treatment strategy on outcomes in patients with candidemia and other forms of invasive candidiasis: a patient-level quantitative review of randomized trials.," *Clinical infectious diseases: an official publication of the Infectious Diseases Society of America*, vol. 54, no. 8, pp. 1110–22, Apr. 2012.

[160] S. García-Sánchez, S. Aubert, I. Iraqui, G. Janbon, J. Ghigo, and C. D'Enfert, "Candida albicans biofilms: a developmental state associated with specific and stable gene expression patterns.," *Eukaryotic cell*, vol. 3, no. 2, pp. 536–45, Apr. 2004.

[161] H. Nailis, D. Vandenbosch, D. Deforce, H. J. Nelis, and T. Coenye, "Transcriptional response to fluconazole and amphotericin B in Candida albicans biofilms.," *Research in microbiology*, vol. 161, no. 4, pp. 284–92, May 2010.

[162] K. Lewis, "Riddle of biofilm resistance.," *Antimicrobial agents and chemotherapy*, vol. 45, no. 4, pp. 999–1007, Apr. 2001.

[163] K. Lewis, "Persister cells.," *Annual review of microbiology*, vol. 64, no. May, pp. 357–72, Jan. 2010.

[164] M. D. LaFleur, C. a Kumamoto, and K. Lewis, "Candida albicans biofilms produce antifungal-tolerant persister cells.," *Antimicrobial agents and chemotherapy*, vol. 50, no. 11, pp. 3839–46, Nov. 2006.

[165] B. Spellberg, A. S. Ibrahim, M. R. Yeaman, L. Lin, Y. Fu, V. Avanesian, A. S. Bayer, S. G. Filler, P. Lipke, H. Otoo, and J. E. Edwards, "The antifungal vaccine derived from the recombinant N terminus of Als3p protects mice against the bacterium Staphylococcus aureus.," *Infection and immunity*, vol. 76, no. 10, pp. 4574–80, Oct. 2008.

[166] B. J. Spellberg, A. S. Ibrahim, V. Avanesian, Y. Fu, C. Myers, Q. T. Phan, S. G. Filler, M. R. Yeaman, and J. E. Edwards, "Efficacy of the anti-Candida rAls3p-N or rAls1p-N vaccines against disseminated and mucosal candidiasis.," *The Journal of infectious diseases*, vol. 194, no. 2, pp. 256–60, Jul. 2006.

[167] S. Sandini, R. La Valle, S. Deaglio, F. Malavasi, A. Cassone, and F. De Bernardis, "A highly immunogenic recombinant and truncated protein of the secreted aspartic proteases family (rSap2t) of Candida albicans as a mucosal anticandidal vaccine.," *FEMS immunology and medical microbiology*, vol. 62, no. 2, pp. 215–24, Jul. 2011.

[168] A. Lepak and D. Andes, "Fungal sepsis: optimizing antifungal therapy in the critical care setting.," *Critical care clinics*, vol. 27, no. 1, pp. 123–47, Jan. 2011.

[169] J. Chahoud, Z. a Kanafani, and S. S. Kanj, "Management of candidaemia and invasive candidiasis in critically ill patients.," *International journal of antimicrobial agents*, May 2013.

[170] P. G. Pappas, C. a Kauffman, D. Andes, D. K. Benjamin, T. F. Calandra, J. E. Edwards, S. G. Filler, J. F. Fisher, B.-J. Kullberg, L. Ostrosky-Zeichner, A. C. Reboli, J. H. Rex, T. J. Walsh, and J. D. Sobel, "Clinical practice guidelines for the management of candidiasis: 2009 update by the Infectious Diseases Society of America.," *Clinical infectious diseases: an official publication of the Infectious Diseases Society of America*, vol. 48, no. 5, pp. 503–35, Mar. 2009.

[171] O. a Cornely, M. Bassetti, T. Calandra, J. Garbino, B. J. Kullberg, O. Lortholary, W. Meersseman, M. Akova, M. C. Arendrup, S. Arikan-Akdagli, J. Bille, E. Castagnola, M. Cuenca-Estrella, J. P. Donnelly, a H. Groll, R. Herbrecht, W. W. Hope, H. E. Jensen, C. Lass-Flörl, G. Petrikkos, M. D. Richardson, E. Roilides, P. E. Verweij, C. Viscoli, and a J. Ullmann, "ESCMID* guideline for the diagnosis and management of Candida diseases 2012: non-neutropenic adult patients.," *Clinical microbiology and infection: the official publication of the European Society of Clinical Microbiology and Infectious Diseases*, vol. 18 Suppl 7, pp. 19–37, Dec. 2012.

[172] W. W. Hope, E. Castagnola, a H. Groll, E. Roilides, M. Akova, M. C. Arendrup, S. Arikan-Akdagli, M. Bassetti, J. Bille, O. a Cornely, M. Cuenca-Estrella, J. P. Donnelly, J. Garbino, R. Herbrecht, H. E. Jensen, B. J. Kullberg, C. Lass-Flörl, O. Lortholary, W. Meersseman, G. Petrikkos, M. D. Richardson, P. E. Verweij, C. Viscoli, and a J. Ullmann, "ESCMID* guideline for the diagnosis and management of Candida diseases 2012: prevention and management of invasive infections in neonates and children caused by Candida spp.," *Clinical microbiology and infection: the official publication of the European Society of Clinical Microbiology and Infectious Diseases*, vol. 18 Suppl 7, pp. 38–52, Dec. 2012.

[173] a J. Ullmann, M. Akova, R. Herbrecht, C. Viscoli, M. C. Arendrup, S. Arikan-Akdagli, M. Bassetti, J. Bille, T. Calandra, E. Castagnola, O. a Cornely, J. P. Donnelly, J. Garbino, a H. Groll, W. W. Hope, H. E. Jensen, B. J. Kullberg, C. Lass-Flörl, O. Lortholary, W. Meersseman, G. Petrikkos, M. D. Richardson, E. Roilides, P. E. Verweij, and M. Cuenca-Estrella, "ESCMID* guideline for the diagnosis and management of Candida diseases 2012: adults with haematological malignancies and after haematopoietic stem cell transplantation (HCT).," *Clinical microbiology and infection: the official publication of the European Society of Clinical Microbiology and Infectious Diseases*, vol. 18 Suppl 7, pp. 53–67, Dec. 2012.

[174] C. J. Walraven and S. a Lee, "Antifungal lock therapy.," *Antimicrobial agents and chemotherapy*, vol. 57, no. 1, pp. 1–8, Jan. 2013.

[175] C. G. Pierce and J. L. Lopez-Ribot, "Candidiasis drug discovery and development: new approaches targeting virulence for discovering and identifying new drugs.," *Expert opinion on drug discovery*, Jun. 2013.

In: Candida *albicans*: Symptoms, Causes and Treatment Options ISBN: 978-1-62808-882-3
Editors: Leon A. Dietrich and Tim S. Friedmann

Chapter II

New Developments in the Pathogenesis of *Candida albicans*: Characterization of Secreted Aspartic Proteases and Profiling of Survival Mechanism in Blood

***Wataru Aoki*[1,2,3] *and Mitsuyoshi Ueda*[2,*]**

[1]Japan Society for the Promotion of Science, Sakyo-ku, Kyoto, Japan
[2]Division of Applied Life Sciences, Graduate School of Agriculture, Kyoto University, Sakyo-ku, Kyoto, Japan
[3]Department of Applied Physics, Division of Precision Science and Applied Physics, Graduate School of Engineering, Osaka University, Suita, Osaka, Japan

Abstract

Candida albicans generally exists as a commensal organism and is present in approximately 50% of the human population. However, if host immunity is compromised, for example by AIDS, immunosuppressive drugs, or cancer chemotherapy, *C. albicans* can opportunistically cause recurrent candidiasis. In particular, the mortality rate from systemic candidiasis is very high due to a lack of effective diagnosis and treatment. Hence, there is an urgent need for clear elucidation of the virulence mechanisms of *C. albicans*.

Degradation of host tissues, evasion of the immune system, and dissemination via the blood stream are integral features of the overall virulence of *C. albicans*, and have been important areas of research. Among virulence factors of *C. albicans* that contribute to these processes, secreted aspartic proteases (Saps) are well-studied enzymes, and their roles have been evaluated in numerous investigations. Recent papers reveal

* Tel: +81-(0)75-753-6110; Fax: +81-(0)75-753-6112; E-mail: miueda@kais.kyoto-u.ac.jp.

unconventional properties of Saps and describe their roles in attacking host cells, degradation of host tissues, and immunity evasion.

In addition to research concentrating on individual attributes, such as Saps, 'omics' approaches offer promising avenues to shed light on the complex virulence processes mentioned above. Analyses of overall virulence processes by omics technologies, for example proteomics, are beginning to uncover novel virulence attributes of *C. albicans*.

This review describes new developments in the characterization of secreted aspartic proteases (Saps) and profiling of virulence processes by proteomics.

Keywords: *Candida albicans*, secreted aspartic protease (Sap), proteome, serum

1. Secreted Aspartic Proteases in Virulence of *C. Albicans*

Ten types of secreted aspartic proteases (Saps1–10) have received particular attention as major virulence attributes of *C. albicans* [1-3], and elucidation of their full functional repertoire has been an important research area. The Sap family is characteristic of the *Candida* genus; *Saccharomyces cerevisiae*, a closely related species, does not have any homologous proteases [4]. Many reports have shown that Sap-deficient *C. albicans* mutants have attenuated virulence [5-11], and it is evident that Sap isozymes have important roles in the infectious processes of *C. albicans*.

Among the ten types of Sap isozymes, Saps1–8 are secretory proteins, while Saps9–10 are glycosylphosphatidylinositol (GPI)-anchored proteins [1]. Sap isozymes are differentially regulated during the virulence processes; Saps1–3 may be important for adherence to host cells and degradation of host tissues [6, 12, 13], while Saps4–6 appear to be produced during yeast-hyphae transition and are involved in systemic diseases [14-17].

Saps were originally thought to be typical aspartic proteases, characterized by optimal activity at acidic pH and sensitivity to pepstatin, a hexapeptide protease inhibitor from *Streptomyces* [18]. In addition, they were recognized to have roles in degradation of host proteins to obtain nitrogen, disruption of host tissues, and evasion of immune cells. Here, we review recent papers relating to the Sap family, which report their unconventional characteristics and reveal novel aspects of *C. albicans* virulence.

Regulatory cascade of SAP expression – Surrounding environmental factors dramatically influence production of Sap isozymes. Characterization of mechanisms regulating *SAP* gene expression will lead to understanding of the strategies used by *C. albicans* in adapting to dynamically changing environments within host tissues. Recently, Dabas *et al.* revealed the regulatory network for Sap2p, a major isozyme that functions to degrade host proteins [19]. The authors disrupted *GLN3* and *GAT1*, GATA transcription factors important for the utilization of alternative nitrogen sources [20-23], and found that this led to *C. albicans* growth defects in medium containing bovine serum albumin as the sole nitrogen source [19]. The growth defect could be compensated by expression of *SAP2* with the constitutive *ADH1* promoter. The authors found that Gln3p and Gat1p were necessary for regulation of *STP1*, which is required for expression of *SAP2*. In addition, the control of *SAP2* expression was dependent on the small GTPase, Rhb1p, linking *C. albicans* to target of rapamycin (TOR) signaling, which is involved in the response to nitrogen availability through regulation of *GAT1* and *GLN3* [23-26].

Crystal structures of Sap isozymes – Determination of the structures of Sap isozymes is essential for knowledge of structure-function relationships and design of structure-based inhibitors. However, only the structure of Sap2, the dominant protease, had been studied as complexes with pepstatin A and A-70450 [27, 28]. Recently, Borelli *et al.* presented the X-ray crystal structures of Saps1, 3, and 5 [29, 30] (Figure 1), which are members of two major subfamilies of Sap isozymes (Saps1–3 and Saps4–6). The structure of Sap3 follows the classical aspartic protease fold, similar to Sap2, and its active site is partly covered by an antiparallel β-hairpin, which is common in aspartic proteases and important for inhibitor or substrate binding [31, 32]. Compared to other aspartic proteases, Saps2 and 3 have enlarged and extended binding sites and their structural features identify them as a distinct subfamily. The N-terminal substrate binding site of Sap3 contains only hydrophobic and/or acidic amino acids and its active site retains a strong overall negative charge, suggesting preference for peptides with hydrophobic and/or basic amino acids. Pepstatin A caused a conformational change within the active site flap of Sap3 which closes on binding to this substrate, significantly narrowing the active site region. This flap movement may be important in allowing the formation of hydrogen bonds and hydrophobic interactions between Sap3 and pepstatin A.

Sap5 is important for the invasion of epithelial tissues in the human oral mucosa [33], and a triple deletion of Saps4–6 attenuated *C. albicans* virulence [10]. The crystal structure of Sap5 revealed clear differences from Saps1–3 in its overall electrostatic charge [29] (Figure 1). Positively charged residues surround the active site, which may raise the optimal pH of Sap5 to 5.0, compared to pH 3.5–4.5 for Saps1–3 [5]. The active site cleft itself is similar, with negatively charged and/or hydrophobic amino acids, indicating a preference for basic or hydrophobic amino acids. Despite the highly conserved overall structures of Saps1–3 and 5, Sap5 displayed some different characteristics, including in electrostatic charge, indicating adaptation to the specific environmental conditions in which the isozymes work. As a future direction, it will be interesting to investigate to what extent the structures of Saps7–10 differ to those of Saps1–6.

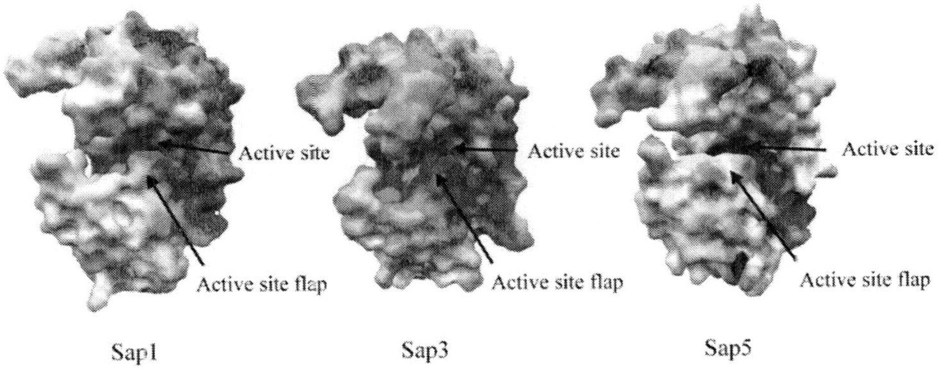

Figure 1. Crystal structures of Saps1, 3, and 5. Negatively charged surface is colored red, and positively charged surface blue. Yellow color indicates hydrophobic residues. These crystal structures are visualized using data from the protein data bank (2QZW, 2H6T, and 2QZX for Sap1, Sap3, and Sap5, respectively).

Using knowledge of the structure of Sap isozymes, inhibitors with broad or narrow specificities can be designed. There is a recent review on protease inhibitors as potential anti-*Candida albicans* drugs [34].

Biochemical properties of Sap isozymes – Sap isozymes can degrade many types of host proteins *in vitro*, including albumin [3], mucin [35], IgG [36], and IgA [37]. In addition, recent studies demonstrate that Saps1–3 can degrade host complement components (C3b, C4b, and C5) and inhibit terminal complement complex formation [38] and that Sap9 can degrade the oral salivary antimicrobial peptide, histatin-5 [39]. These findings suggest that *C. albicans* may evade, not only adaptive immunity, but also the innate immune system. Furthermore, Sap isozymes of *C. albicans* have roles in processing of cell surface proteins to modulate cellular responses. Puri et al. showed that Sap8 potentially served as a major regulator of Msb2p [40], demonstrating that cleavage of this molecule led to release of its extracellular domain, which in turn allowed Cek1p phosphorylation. Cek1p is associated with mitogen activated protein kinase pathways and important for dimorphism, biofilm formation, and virulence [41-43]. It is assumed that the Sap family is also essential for the perception of external stimuli and generation of appropriate responses to these.

Koelsch et al. first showed the biochemical mechanism underlying the degradation of many host proteins by Sap isozymes [18], extending previous study of Sap2 alone [44]; they purified Saps1–3, and 6, and determined their optimal pH and substrate specificities using defined mixtures of peptide substrates. They found that Saps1–3 degraded peptide bonds between large hydrophobic amino acids, and that the details of their broad specificities differed among the four isozymes. Recently, Schild et al. [45] and Albrecht et al. [46] investigated the enzymatic properties of the GPI-anchored proteins, Saps9 and 10. Saps9 and 10 exhibited optimum activity at near neutral pH and preferred to process peptides with basic or dibasic residues, while both proteases also cleaved at non-basic sites. Furthermore, the authors identified covalently linked cell wall proteins, including Cht2p and Pir1p as protease substrates [45]. This result was verified using hemagglutinin epitope-tagged *C. albicans* cells. In addition, deletion of Saps9 and 10 affected cell separation during budding and attenuated epithelial cell damage during experimental oral infection. Thus, Saps9 and 10 could have important roles in cell wall structure and integrity.

Recently, properties of all types of Sap isozymes were comprehensively characterized based on the reports described above [47] (Table 1). Reported optimal pHs of Sap isozymes were broadly distributed between pH 2.5 (Sap8) and pH 6.5 (Sap7). The presence of Sap isozymes functioning within a broad range of optimum pHs may allow *C. albicans* to survive and cause infections in various tissues. The substrate specificities of Sap isozymes were analyzed using fluorescence-quenched peptide libraries consisting of 475 peptides, and P_1 substrate specificities were comprehensively characterized. Saps1–6, and 8 were found to have broad substrate specificities and could cleave peptides with positively charged or large hydrophobic amino acids at the P_1 position, consistent with the previous report [18]. In contrast, Saps7, 9, and 10 showed high substrate specificities and preferred Met, Arg, and His, respectively, at the P_1 site. While Sap7 has been the focus of less experimental attention to date, it has some characteristic features; expression of *SAP7* mRNA is not detected under laboratory growth conditions [48-50], the protein exhibits optimal protease activity at neutral pH [47], and a *SAP7* null mutant shows attenuated virulence in an intravenous mouse model of infection [51]. In addition, Sap7 was found to be a pepstatin A-insensitive protease; the amino acid composition around the active site might affect the accessibility of pepstatin A

[52] and Saps9 and 10 are not completely inhibited by pepstatin A [45]. These observations may explain the lack of a significant effect of pepstatin A on virulence of *C. albicans* in some infection models [53, 54].

Table 1. Biochemical properties of Sap isozymes

Isozyme name	Sap1	Sap2	Sap3	Sap4	Sap5	Sap6	Sap7	Sap8	Sap9	Sap10
Theoretical molecular mass (k)	36	36	37	37	37	37	47	35	53	45
Apparent molecular mass (k)	39	38	37	39	36	38	52 and 15	36	44 and 11	42
N-linked glycosylation*1	-	-	-	+	-	+	+	+	+	+
Optimum pH	5.0	4.0	3.0	5.0	5.0	5.0	5.5	2.5	5.5	6.0
Pepstatin A sensitivity*2	+	+	+	+	+	+	-	+	+	+

*1 +, glycosylated; -, non-glycosylated.
*2 +, sensitive to peptstatin A; -, insensitive to pepstatin A.

Virulence roles of Sap isozymes – The sap family is important for tissue damage [1, 6], however, the invasive mechanism is not yet fully understood. In this section, we review recent reports that have succeeded in shedding light on the physiological roles of Sap isozymes.

Villar et al. found that E-cadherin of host cells was degraded at the site of *C. albicans* invasion of oral epithelial tissues [33] and invasion deficient *C. albicans rim101/rim101* showed decreased degradation of E-cadherin, probably dependent on low expression of *SAPs4–6*. Indeed, engineered expression of *SAP5* restored degradation of E-cadherin in this strain [33]. Other reports have shown that the Sap family can degrade human Laminin-332, a component of basement membrane [55]. These reports suggest the importance of the proteolytic activities of Sap isozymes in the degradation of adherence junctions [56].

Sap isozymes may contribute to the induction of an inflammatory response by the host immune system [57-59]. A recent report on interactions between host and *C. albicans* revealed that Sap9 had a major role in the recognition of *C. albicans* cells by polymorphonuclear neutrophils (PMNs) [60]. Sap9 was required for the induction of chemotaxis and the release of reactive oxygen intermediates of PMNs. Alterations in the processing of cell surface proteins by Saps9 and 10 may alter the immunogenicity of *C. albicans*. Research in the field of cytokines, has shown that *C. albicans* induced the production of interleukin 1α (IL-1α), IL-1β, IL-6, IL-8, IL-10, granulocyte-macrophage colony-stimulating factor, gamma interferon, and tumor necrosis factor alpha in a reconstituted human vaginal epithelium (RHVE) model [61]. Pepstatin A strongly reduced the cytokine response, and *SAP1*- or *SAP2*-null mutants reduced tissue damage and cytokine production, indicating an association between the Sap family and the proinflammatory cytokine response [61]. However, inhibition of Sap isozymes by pepstatin A did not completely account for the induced cytokine production, indicating other *C. albicans*-mediated proinflammatory mechanisms. Recently, Pietrella et al. reported that recombinant

Saps1–3 and 6 significantly induced cytokine production in human monocytes [62]. Treatment with pepstatin A did not affect cytokine secretion, and the stimulatory potential of Sap isozymes was independent of protease-activated receptor activation in human monocytes. The inflammatory response was shown to be partially dependent on the denaturation of Sap isozymes. Sap isozymes could induce an inflammatory response without proteolytic activities, suggesting an activity-independent response to Sap isozymes [62]. A very recent report by Pietrella et al. found that Sap2 and Sap6 induced cytokine production through inflammasome activation [63]. This phenomenon occurred via NLRP3 (NOD-like receptor family, pyrin domain containing 3) and caspase-1 activation, which led to maturation of IL-1β, a cytokine induced by Sap isozymes in monocytes. The process required internalization of Sap isozymes via a clathrin-dependent pathway. Hence, Sap isozymes may contribute to the virulence of *C. albicans* by fostering host immunity.

Inflammatory cytokine responses could be dependent on inter-strain genetic diversity of *C. albicans*. Some papers have reported the possibility of associations between clusters of genetically related *C. albicans* strains and infectious ability at different anatomical sites [64], probably due to differences in adhesion, degradation, and invasion abilities. Whiley et al. investigated differences in the cytokine responses of epithelial cells, and showed considerable variation in site-specificity and induction profiles of cytokines using two oral and two vaginal reference strains of *C. albicans* [65]. The NCPF8112 strain, from a patient with recurrent episodes of vaginal candidiasis, with the highest detectable levels of Sap isozymes, did not elicit a response from either oral or vaginal epithelial models, indicating the existence of additional proinflammatory factors. Correlation between proinflammatory responses and levels of phospholipase activity in *C. albicans* has been also suggested [65].

An unusual function of the Sap family, identified by Wu et al., is that Saps4–6 cause apoptotis of epithelial cells by a novel Trojan horse mechanism [66]. Through induction of apoptosis, Saps4–6 containing RGD/KGD motifs bound to integrins of epithelial cells and were internalized in endosomes. This internalization induced permeabilization of lysosomes and triggered apoptosis via caspase activation. RGD-containing peptides inhibited this process, and Sap4–6 mutants, lacking RGD/KGD motifs, were ineffective in triggering apoptosis, indicating the importance of interactions between integrins and Sap isozymes.

Expression profiles of the SAP gene family – Investigation of the expression profiles of the *SAP* gene family during the course of infection has been an important research area for clarification of the association between Sap isozymes and the virulence of *C. albicans* [6, 14, 67]. Taylor et al. investigated expression profiles of *SAPs1–6* using *in vivo* expression technology (IVET), which enables detection of transient gene expression at the single-cell level during vaginal infection in mouse [68]. Among *SAPs1–6*, only *SAP4* and *SAP5* were detectably induced during infection of the mouse model and expression of *SAPs4–6* were associated with hyphal growth. *SAP5* was expressed in 48 ± 10% of fungal cells soon after infection, while *SAP4* was expressed in 25 ± 10% of fungal cells at later stages, indicating strict temporal regulation of gene expression patterns. In the previous study, different expression patterns of the *SAP* gene family in other expression models were observed by RT-PCR or IVET [6, 49, 69]. For example, it was shown that *SAP5* and *SAP6* but not *SAP4* were expressed in the esophageal epithelium [70]. These observations suggested that each Sap isozyme might play a specific role in various infection models. Lian et al. also investigated expression profiles of *SAPs1–7* in asymptomatic *Candida* carriage and women with vulvovaginal candidiasis using RT-PCR [48]. *SAPs2*, *4–6*, and *7* were found to be expressed in both groups, and *SAP1* and *SAP3* transcripts were observed only in the patient group. Further investigation of various human candidiasis will be important to reveal correlation between expression profiles of the *SAP* gene family and types of candidiasis.

Rethinking of the physiological roles of the Sap family – The many studies discussed above have contributed to clarification of the roles of the Sap family in the pathogenesis of superficial and disseminated candidiasis. However, some reports have forced us to rethink the importance of the Sap family in some models [11, 53, 54, 71]. Naglik et al. investigated the expression profiles of *SAP* genes using RT-PCR to identify which contributed to candidiasis infection of human epithelium *in vitro* and *in vivo* [71]. The contribution of *SAPs1–3* and *SAPs4–6* appeared to be low in organotypic RHE (reconstituted human epithelium) models, whereas *SAP5* and *SAP9* were significantly expressed *in vivo* and *SAP5* was the only gene upregulated during infection progression. In addition, pepstatin A reduced tissue damage in these models, suggesting roles for the Sap family in epithelial infection; however, hyphal formation itself appeared to be the major cause of tissue damage, since hyphae-deficient mutants demonstrated significantly reduced virulence of *C. albicans*, despite normal expression of *SAP5*. Lermann et al. also reported that *SAP5* alone was detectably expressed in *in vitro* RHE models, and that *C. albicans* mutants lacking all of the *SAPs1–3* or *SAPs4–6* genes showed the same capacity to invade RHE models as the wild-type strain [53]. These observations indicated a low contribution of the Sap family in superficial infection models; however, F. C. Odds pointed out that these studies used the *C. albicans* strain SC5314, which has been well known to be poor at colonizing and invading mammalian epithelia *in vivo* [11, 72]. Moreover, the roles of Saps7–10 were not investigated. Thus, further investigation is justified.

More recently, Correia et al. reassessed the roles of *SAPs1–6* in a murine model of hematogenously disseminated candidiasis, using a *C. albicans sap*-null mutant unaffected by *URA3* expression. While URA-blaster is a convenient technique to construct *C. albicans* mutants [73], this method can lead to a misinterpretation of results regarding *C. albicans* virulence, due to ectopic expression of the *URA3* marker. [74-77]. The authors found that virulence of *C. albicans* lacking *SAPs1–3* was equivalent to that of the wild type strain, *C. albicans* SC5314, and that a mutant lacking *SAP5* displayed slightly less virulence. This result suggested a limited role for Saps1–6 in murine hematogenously disseminated candidiasis. In addition, Dunkel et al. showed that loss of heterozygosity at an unlinked genomic locus might be responsible for the phenotype of a *C. albicans SAPs4–6* mutant in previous studies [78]. Further investigation of the virulence of *C. albicans* will need to solve these technical problems by developing a novel technique to construct *C. albicans* mutants not affected by ectopic expression of selective markers or loss of heterozygosity.

2. Profiling of Proteome Variations in *C. Albicans*

Virulence processes of *C. albicans*, such as degradation of host tissues, evasion from immune cells, resistance to drugs, and adaptation to blood serum are highly complex; the traditional virulence attributes, including Saps, adhesins, and yeast-hyphal transition cannot fully explain overall virulence, and the existence of other unknown contributing factors is anticipated. Completion of the sequencing of the *C. albicans* genome provides an opportunity to analyze these complicated processes. In particular, proteome analysis is a promising method to reveal the mysteries of *C. albicans*, as this technique could directly detect virulence effectors on a global scale. Transcriptome analysis is an alternative approach to reveal dynamic variations [79, 80], however, a number of studies have indicated that the correlation between the transcriptome and the proteome in eukaryotic cells is weak [81, 82]. Proteome analysis that precisely reflects the abundance of proteins will be an important approach to reveal virulence factors of *Candida albicans*.

Two-dimensional polyacrylamide gel electrophoresis (2D-PAGE) is a major technique in the analysis of proteome dynamics. In addition, the application of liquid chromatography-tandem mass spectrometry (LC-MS/MS) enables the identification of proteins that are difficult to separate by 2D-PAGE because of hydrophobicity, low abundance, extreme pI, or molecular mass. Using these technologies, proteome analyses have been applied to investigate responses against deprivation of amino acid [83] and nitrogen [22], exchange of carbon-sources [84], and drug administration [85]. There are previous excellent reviews on proteome research [86-88]. Here we review recent proteome reports relating to survival in blood that is an essential part of the virulence of *C. albicans* in producing systemic infections.

Methodologies for proteome analysis – For proteome analysis, it is important to select the optimal methodology according to the specific purpose of the study. Many types of proteome methodologies, consisting of a separation technique in combination with mass spectrometry, have been developed [89]. Among these, there are two major methodologies for proteome analysis: gel-based proteomics using 2D-PAGE and shotgun proteomics with LC-MS/MS [90]. 2D-PAGE is the most popular technique for separation of proteins according to their isoelectric points (pI) and molecular mass. This robust technique can separate thousands of proteins and detect spots at the nanogram level by silver staining. However, gel-to-gel variation in 2D-PAGE can cause difficulties in comparisons to assess differences between several proteome samples. Two-dimensional difference gel electrophoresis (2D-DIGE) is a more powerful technique than 2D-PAGE. In this technique, up to three proteome samples are labeled with fluorescent dyes and applied to the same gel, reducing experimental variation. The 2D-DIGE technology is a robust and sensitive method for the detection of proteins at the low nanogram level. The disadvantages of these gel-based technologies are low-throughput, low identification rate, and limitations of separation factors.

Shotgun proteomics is a promising, alternative way to identify a large number of proteins, including scarce proteins, in a high-throughput manner. By using this system, it is even possible to identify femtomolar level proteins, which are difficult to identify in gel-based proteomics. The technique has advantages in comprehensiveness and identification rates, however, there are some limitations with a complex proteome samples, due to ionization suppression. Though many mechanisms of ionization suppression have been proposed, high analyte concentrations, due to insufficient separation, reduce the efficiency of ionization, leading to poor identification rates.

A system using ultra-performance chromatographic separation with a monolithic column could reduce ionization suppression and has shown excellent performance in protein identification (Figure 2). A monolithic silica column, prepared from a mixture of tetramethoxysilane and methyltrimethoxysilane in a long-fused silica capillary [91], showed higher separation performance than the conventional particle-packed columns [92]. Higher separation leads to low ionization suppression, enabling identification of several thousands of proteins in a single analysis. For example, a system using a long monolithic silica capillary column (350 cm) successfully identified 2602 proteins produced in *Escherichia coli* cells in a one-shot analysis [93]. In addition, the recent development of various types of stable isotope labeling will be powerful tools in improving quantification efficiency [94].

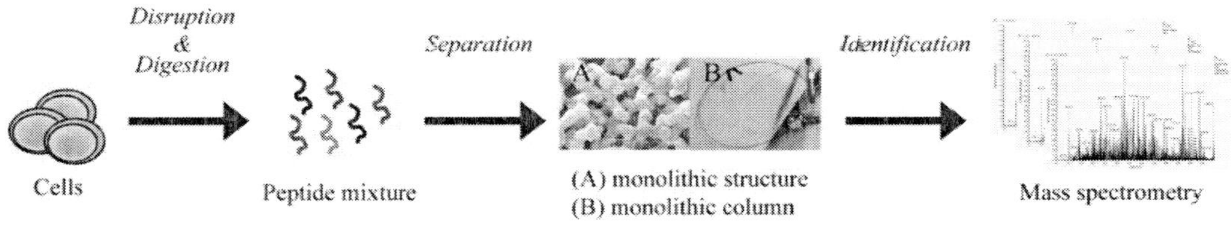

Figure 2. Shotgun proteomics using a long monolithic silica capillary column. The monolithic column allows better separation, leading to efficient identification of thousands of proteins.

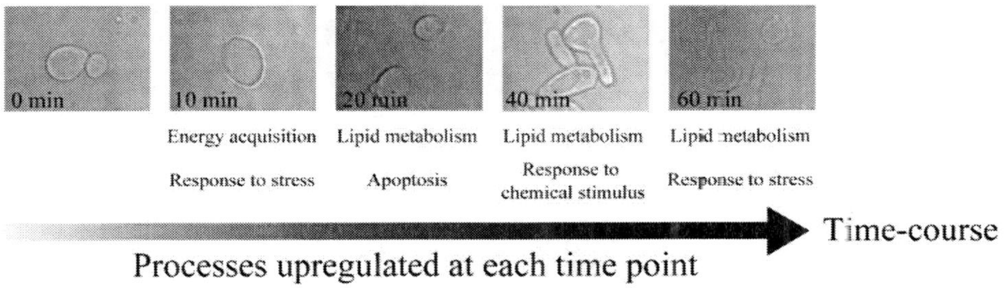

Figure 3. Representation of the results of time-course proteomics.

Identification of potential virulence factors of C. albicans for adaptation to a serum – Hyphal extension is a major characteristic of *C. albicans* under serum conditions. Klis et al. investigated changes in the wall proteome during hyphal extension using Fourier transform-MS combined with ^{15}N-metabolically labeled reference culture [95]. They used 3 hyphal induction methods; fetal calf serum, *N*-acetylglucosamine, and Iscove's modified Dulbecco's medium and quantified 21 cell-wall proteins. The three induction methods caused similar proteome changes, all strongly inducing levels of Als3p, Hwp2p, Hyr1p, Plb5p, and Sod5p incorporation, proteins known as important virulence factors. Thus, these factors could be indicators of hyphal growth. By contrast, levels of Rhd3p, Sod4p, and Ywp1p were strongly decreased, and these proteins were shown to be indicators of yeast morphology. In addition, the authors remarked that these wall proteins could be promising targets for vaccine development, since the cell surface is exposed to outer environments. Indeed, vaccination with Als3p [96] or Hyr1p [97] showed protective effects after injection of *C. albicans*.

Recently, time-course variations of the *C. albicans* proteome during recognition of a blood serum were revealed by shotgun proteomics [98]. In almost all previous reports, endpoint samples of cells incubated for several hours were used for proteome analyses [99-101]. Thus, this study can be thought of as a complementary approach, and will provide insights into the strategy of *C. albicans* for adaptation to the serum. In an attempt to carry out time-course proteomics, high-throughput proteome analysis was performed using a LC-MS/MS system with a long monolithic silica capillary column. Using this system, the early stage of adaptation to the serum was analyzed. These conditions may partially reflect the behavior of *C. albicans* during initial systemic candidiasis, a process in which *C. albicans* recognizes the blood stream, adapts to the conditions therein, and metastasizes to organs. *C. albicans* was cultivated in fetal bovine serum, and 1,418 proteins were identified in endpoint samples incubated for 0 or 60 min. Among these, 16 proteins were identified by time-course analysis as nascent/newly synthesized proteins during adaptation to the serum, and are candidates as important factors in serum adaption (Table 2). Gene ontology analysis revealed that the 16 proteins were enriched for transport-related proteins, indicating that *C. albicans* probably first prioritizes the acquisition of essential elements (Figure 3). This approach will be refined using quantitative analysis that can capture dynamic variations of proteome. Such research could identify important virulence factors, leading to the development of novel pharmaceuticals.

Table 2. Candidate factors important for serum adaption

ORF No.	Description	Candida GO-Slim Process
orf19.5437	RHR2; Glycerol 3-phosphatase	Response to stress; Carbohydrate metabolic process
orf19.4527	HGT1; High-affinity glucose transporter	Transport; Response to chemical stimulus; Response to drug
orf19.3767	Not characterized; Ortholog(s) have role in protein targeting to vacuole	Transport; Protein catabolic process
orf19.7678	ATP16; Subunit of the mitochondrial F1F0 ATP synthase	Transport
orf19.713	Not characterized; Ortholog(s) have role in apoptosis	Biological process unknown
orf19.3686	Not characterized; Ortholog(s) have role in mitochondrial proton-transporting ATP synthase complex assembly	Organelle organization
orf19.487	SPT14; Putative DNA-binding transcription factor	Lipid metabolic process; Protein modification process
orf19.4825	Not characterized	Biological process unknown
orf19.1631	ERG6; Delta(24)-sterol C-methyltransferase	Response to chemical stimulus; Lipid metabolic process; Response to drug
orf19.4620	Not characterized; Ortholog(s) have role in protein import into mitochondrial inner membrane	Transport; Organelle organization; Cellular membrane organization
orf19.4594	Not characterized; Ortholog(s) have role in endocytosis	Transport; Cellular membrane organization; Vesicle-mediated transport
orf19.5342.2	Not characterized	Biological process unknown
orf19.4123	Not characterized; Putative THO complex subunit	Transport; Response to stress; RNA metabolic process; DNA metabolic process
orf19.2439	Not characterized	Lipid metabolic process
orf19.6211	Not characterized	Biological process unknown
orf19.2009	PEX12; Ortholog(s) have role in protein import into peroxisome matrix	Transport; Organelle organization

References

[1] Schaller, M., Borelli, C., Korting, H.C., and Hube, B. (2005). Hydrolytic enzymes as virulence factors of *Candida albicans*. *Mycoses,* 48, 365-377.

[2] Naglik, J., Albrecht, A., Bader, O., and Hube, B. (2004). *Candida albicans* proteinases and host/pathogen interactions. *Cell Microbiol.,* 6, 915-926.

[3] Naglik, J.R., Challacombe, S.J., and Hube, B. (2003). *Candida albicans* secreted aspartyl proteinases in virulence and pathogenesis. *Microbiol. Mol. Biol. Rev.* 67, 400-428.

[4] Parra-Ortega, B., Cruz-Torres, H., Villa-Tanaca, L., and Hernandez-Rodriguez, C. (2009). Phylogeny and evolution of the aspartyl protease family from clinically relevant *Candida* species. *Mem. Inst. Oswaldo Cruz,* 104, 505-512.

[5] Borg-von Zepelin, M., Beggah, S., Boggian, K., Sanglard, D., and Monod, M. (1998). The expression of the secreted aspartyl proteinases Sap4 to Sap6 from *Candida albicans* in murine macrophages. *Mol. Microbiol.,* 28, 543-554.

[6] Schaller, M., Bein, M., Korting, H.C., Baur, S., Hamm, G., Monod, M., Beinhauer, S., and Hube, B. (2003). The secreted aspartyl proteinases Sap1 and Sap2 cause tissue damage in an *in vitro* model of vaginal candidiasis based on reconstituted human vaginal epithelium. *Infect. Immun.,* 71, 3227-3234.

[7] Fallon, K., Bausch, K., Noonan, J., Huguenel, E., and Tamburini, P. (1997). Role of aspartic proteases in disseminated *Candida albicans* infection in mice. *Infect. Immun.,* 65, 551-556.

[8] De Bernardis, F., Boccanera, M., Adriani, D., Spreghini, E., Santoni, G., and Cassone, A. (1997). Protective role of antimannan and anti-aspartyl proteinase antibodies in an experimental model of *Candida albicans* vaginitis in rats. *Infect. Immun.,* 65, 3399-3405.

[9] Hube, B. (1998). Possible role of secreted proteinases in *Candida albicans* infections. *Rev. Iberoam. Micol.,* 15, 65-68.

[10] Sanglard, D., Hube, B., Monod, M., Odds, F.C., and Gow, N.A. (1997). A triple deletion of the secreted aspartyl proteinase genes *SAP4*, *SAP5*, and *SAP6* of *Candida albicans* causes attenuated virulence. *Infect. Immun.,* 65, 3539-3546.

[11] Odds, F.C. (2008). Secreted proteinases and *Candida albicans* virulence. *Microbiology,* 154, 3245-3246.

[12] De Bernardis, F., Cassone, A., Sturtevant, J., and Calderone, R. (1995). Expression of *Candida albicans SAP1* and *SAP2* in experimental vaginitis. *Infect. Immun.,* 63, 1887-1892.

[13] Schaller, M., Hube, B., Ollert, M.W., Schafer, W., Borg-von Zepelin, M., Thoma-Greber, E., and Korting, H.C. (1999). *In vivo* expression and localization of *Candida albicans* secreted aspartyl proteinases during oral candidiasis in HIV-infected patients. *J. Invest. Dermatol.,* 112, 383-386.

[14] Hube, B., Monod, M., Schofield, D.A., Brown, A.J., and Gow, N.A. (1994). Expression of seven members of the gene family encoding secretory aspartyl proteinases in *Candida albicans*. *Mol. Microbiol.,* 14, 87-99.

[15] Schaller, M., Korting, H.C., Schafer, W., Bastert, J., Chen, W., and Hube, B. (1999). Secreted aspartic proteinase (Sap) activity contributes to tissue damage in a model of human oral candidosis. *Mol. Microbiol.,* 34, 169-180.

[16] Tavanti, A., Pardini, G., Campa, D., Davini, P., Lupetti, A., and Senesi, S. (2004). Differential expression of secretory aspartyl proteinase genes (*SAP1-10*) in oral *Candida albicans* isolates with distinct karyotypes. *J. Clin. Microbiol.,* 42, 4726-4734.

[17] Ripeau, J.S., Fiorillo, M., Aumont, F., Belhumeur, P., and de Repentigny, L. (2002). Evidence for differential expression of *Candida albicans* virulence genes during oral infection in intact and human immunodeficiency virus type 1-transgenic mice. *J. Infect. Dis.,* 185, 1094-1102.

[18] Koelsch, G., Tang, J., Loy, J.A., Monod, M., Jackson, K., Foundling, S.I., and Lin, X. (2000). Enzymic characteristics of secreted aspartic proteases of *Candida albicans. Biochim. Biophys. Acta.,* 1480, 117-131.

[19] Dabas, N., and Morschhauser, J. (2008). A transcription factor regulatory cascade controls secreted aspartic protease expression in *Candida albicans. Mol. Microbiol.,* 69, 586-602.

[20] Limjindaporn, T., Khalaf, R.A., and Fonzi, W.A. (2003). Nitrogen metabolism and virulence of *Candida albicans* require the GATA-type transcriptional activator encoded by GAT1. *Mol. Microbiol.,* 50, 993-1004.

[21] Dabas, N., and Morschhauser, J. (2007). Control of ammonium permease expression and filamentous growth by the GATA transcription factors *GLN3* and *GAT1* in *Candida albicans. Eukaryot. Cell,* 6, 875-888.

[22] Morschhauser, J. (2011). Nitrogen regulation of morphogenesis and protease secretion in *Candida albicans. Int. J. Med. Microbiol.,* 301, 390-394.

[23] Liao, W.L., Ramon, A.M., and Fonzi, W.A. (2008). *GLN3* encodes a global regulator of nitrogen metabolism and virulence of *C. albicans. Fungal. Genet. Biol.,* 45, 514-526.

[24] Chen, Y.T., Lin, C.Y., Tsai, P.W., Yang, C.Y., Hsieh, W.P., and Lan, C.Y. (2011). Rhb1 regulates the expression of secreted aspartic protease 2 through the TOR signaling pathway in *Candida albicans. Eukaryot. Cell,* 11, 168-182.

[25] Beck, T., and Hall, M.N. (1999). The TOR signalling pathway controls nuclear localization of nutrient-regulated transcription factors. *Nature,* 402, 689-692.

[26] Kuruvilla, F.G., Shamji, A.F., and Schreiber, S.L. (2001). Carbon- and nitrogen-quality signaling to translation are mediated by distinct GATA-type transcription factors. *Proc. Natl. Acad. Sci. USA,* 98, 7283-7288.

[27] Cutfield, S., Marshall, C., Moody, P., Sullivan, P., and Cutfield, J. (1993). Crystallization of inhibited aspartic proteinase from *Candida albicans. J. Mol. Biol.,* 234, 1266-1269.

[28] Cutfield, S.M., Dodson, E.J., Anderson, B.F., Moody, P.C., Marshall, C.J., Sullivan, P.A., and Cutfield, J.F. (1995). The crystal structure of a major secreted aspartic proteinase from *Candida albicans* in complexes with two inhibitors. *Structure,* 3, 1261-1271.

[29] Borelli, C., Ruge, E., Lee, J.H., Schaller, M., Vogelsang, A., Monod, M., Korting, H.C., Huber, R., and Maskos, K. (2008). X-ray structures of Sap1 and Sap5: structural comparison of the secreted aspartic proteinases from *Candida albicans. Proteins,* 72, 1308-1319.

[30] Borelli, C., Ruge, E., Schaller, M., Monod, M., Korting, H.C., Huber, R., and Maskos, K. (2007). The crystal structure of the secreted aspartic proteinase 3 from *Candida albicans* and its complex with pepstatin A. *Proteins,* 68, 738-748.

[31] Abad-Zapatero, C., Goldman, R., Muchmore, S.W., Hutchins, C., Stewart, K., Navaza, J., Payne, C.D., and Ray, T.L. (1996). Structure of a secreted aspartic protease from *C. albicans* complexed with a potent inhibitor: implications for the design of antifungal agents. *Protein. Sci.,* 5, 640-652.

[32] Davies, D.R. (1990). The structure and function of the aspartic proteinases. *Annu. Rev. Biophys. Biophys. Chem.,* 19, 189-215.

[33] Villar, C.C., Kashleva, H., Nobile, C.J., Mitchell, A.P., and Dongari-Bagtzoglou, A. (2007). Mucosal tissue invasion by *Candida albicans* is associated with E-cadherin degradation, mediated by transcription factor Rim101p and protease Sap5p. *Infect. Immun.,* 75, 2126-2135.

[34] Braga-Silva, L.A., and Santos, A.L. (2011). Aspartic protease inhibitors as potential anti-*Candida albicans* drugs: impacts on fungal biology, virulence and pathogenesis. *Curr. Med. Chem.,* 18, 2401-2419.

[35] Colina, A.R., Aumont, F., Deslauriers, N., Belhumeur, P., and de Repentigny, L. (1996). Evidence for degradation of gastrointestinal mucin by *Candida albicans* secretory aspartyl proteinase. *Infect. Immun.,* 64, 4514-4519.

[36] Kaminishi, H., Miyaguchi, H., Tamaki, T., Suenaga, N., Hisamatsu, M., Mihashi, I., Matsumoto, H., Maeda, H., and Hagihara, Y. (1995). Degradation of humoral host defense by *Candida albicans* proteinase. *Infect. Immun.,* 63, 984-988.

[37] Ruchel, R. (1986). Cleavage of immunoglobulins by pathogenic yeasts of the genus *Candida. Microbiol. Sci.,* 3, 316-319.

[38] Gropp, K., Schild, L., Schindler, S., Hube, B., Zipfel, P.F., and Skerka, C. (2009). The yeast *Candida albicans* evades human complement attack by secretion of aspartic proteases. *Mol. Immunol.,* 47, 465-475.

[39] Meiller, T.F., Hube, B., Schild, L., Shirtliff, M.E., Scheper, M.A., Winkler, R., Ton, A., and Jabra-Rizk, M.A. (2009). A novel immune evasion strategy of *Candida albicans*: proteolytic cleavage of a salivary antimicrobial peptide. *PLoS ONE,* 4, e5039.

[40] Puri, S., Kumar, R., Chadha, S., Tati, S., Conti, H.R., Hube, B., Cullen, P.J., and Edgerton, M. (2012). Secreted aspartic protease cleavage of *Candida albicans* Msb2 activates Cek1 MAPK signaling affecting biofilm formation and oropharyngeal candidiasis. *PLoS ONE,* 7, e46020.

[41] Monge, R.A., Roman, E., Nombela, C., and Pla, J. (2006). The MAP kinase signal transduction network in *Candida albicans*. *Microbiology,* 152, 905-912.

[42] Csank, C., Schroppel, K., Leberer, E., Harcus, D., Mohamed, O., Meloche, S., Thomas, D.Y., and Whiteway, M. (1998). Roles of the *Candida albicans* mitogen-activated protein kinase homolog, Cek1p, in hyphal development and systemic candidiasis. *Infect. .Immun.,* 66, 2713-2721.

[43] Roman, E., Cottier, F., Ernst, J.F., and Pla, J. (2009). Msb2 signaling mucin controls activation of Cek1 mitogen-activated protein kinase in *Candida albicans*. *Eukaryot. Cell,* 8, 1235-1249.

[44] Fusek, M., Smith, E.A., Monod, M., Dunn, B.M., and Foundling, S.I. (1994). Extracellular aspartic proteinases from *Candida albicans*, *Candida tropicalis*, and

Candida parapsilosis yeasts differ substantially in their specificities. *Biochemistry,* 33, 9791-9799.

[45] Schild, L., Heyken, A., de Groot, P.W., Hiller, E., Mock, M., de Koster, C., Horn, U., Rupp, S., and Hube, B. (2011). Proteolytic cleavage of covalently linked cell wall proteins by *Candida albicans* Sap9 and Sap10. *Eukaryot. Cell,* 10, 98-109.

[46] Albrecht, A., Felk, A., Pichova, I., Naglik, J.R., Schaller, M., de Groot, P., Maccallum, D., Odds, F.C., Schafer, W., Klis, F., et al. (2006). Glycosylphosphatidylinositol-anchored proteases of *Candida albicans* target proteins necessary for both cellular processes and host-pathogen interactions. *J. Biol. Chem.,* 281, 688-694.

[47] Aoki, W., Kitahara, N., Miura, N., Morisaka, H., Yamamoto, Y., Kuroda, K., and Ueda, M. (2011). Comprehensive characterization of secreted aspartic proteases encoded by a virulence gene family in *Candida albicans*. *J. Biochem.,* 150, 431-438.

[48] Lian, C.H., and Liu, W.D. (2007). Differential expression of *Candida albicans* secreted aspartyl proteinase in human vulvovaginal candidiasis. *Mycoses,* 50, 383-390.

[49] Naglik, J.R., Rodgers, C.A., Shirlaw, P.J., Dobbie, J.L., Fernandes-Naglik, L.L., Greenspan, D., Agabian, N., and Challacombe, S.J. (2003). Differential expression of *Candida albicans* secreted aspartyl proteinase and phospholipase B genes in humans correlates with active oral and vaginal infections. *J. Infect. Dis.,* 188, 469-479.

[50] Naglik, J.R., Newport, G., White, T.C., Fernandes-Naglik, L.L., Greenspan, J.S., Greenspan, D., Sweet, S.P., Challacombe, S.J., and Agabian, N. (1999). *In vivo* analysis of secreted aspartyl proteinase expression in human oral candidiasis. *Infect. Immun.,* 67, 2482-2490.

[51] Taylor, B.N., Hannemann, H., Sehnal, M., Biesemeier, A., Schweizer, A., Rollinghoff, M., and Schroppel, K. (2005). Induction of *SAP7* correlates with virulence in an intravenous infection model of candidiasis but not in a vaginal infection model in mice. *Infect. Immun.,* 73, 7061-7063.

[52] Aoki, W., Kitahara, N., Miura, N., Morisaka, H., Yamamoto, Y., Kuroda, K., and Ueda, M. (2012). *Candida albicans* possesses Sap7 as a pepstatin A-insensitive secreted aspartic protease. *PLoS ONE,* 7, e32513.

[53] Lermann, U., and Morschhauser, J. (2008). Secreted aspartic proteases are not required for invasion of reconstituted human epithelia by *Candida albicans*. *Microbiology,* 154, 3281-3295.

[54] Kretschmar, M., Felk, A., Staib, P., Schaller, M., Hess, D., Callapina, M., Morschhauser, J., Schafer, W., Korting, H.C., Hof, H., et al. (2002). Individual acid aspartic proteinases (Saps) 1-6 of *Candida albicans* are not essential for invasion and colonization of the gastrointestinal tract in mice. *Microb. Pathog.,* 32, 61-70.

[55] Parnanen, P., Kari, K., Virtanen, I., Sorsa, T., and Meurman, J.H. (2008). Human laminin-332 degradation by *Candida* proteinases. *J. Oral. Pathol. Med.,* 37, 329-335.

[56] Parnanen, P., Meurman, J.H., Samaranayake, L., and Virtanen, I. (2010). Human oral keratinocyte E-cadherin degradation by *Candida albicans* and *Candida glabrata*. *J. Oral. Pathol. Med.,* 39, 275-278.

[57] Beausejour, A., Grenier, D., Goulet, J.P., and Deslauriers, N. (1998). Proteolytic activation of the interleukin-1beta precursor by *Candida albicans*. *Infect. Immun.,* 66, 676-681.

[58] Schaller, M., Mailhammer, R., Grassl, G., Sander, C.A., Hube, B., and Korting, H.C. (2002). Infection of human oral epithelia with *Candida* species induces cytokine expression correlated to the degree of virulence. *J. Invest. Dermatol.,* 118, 652-657.

[59] Steele, C., and Fidel, P.L., Jr. (2002). Cytokine and chemokine production by human oral and vaginal epithelial cells in response to *Candida albicans*. *Infect. Immun.,* 70, 577-583.

[60] Hornbach, A., Heyken, A., Schild, L., Hube, B., Loffler, J., and Kurzai, O. (2009). The glycosylphosphatidylinositol-anchored protease Sap9 modulates the interaction of *Candida albicans* with human neutrophils. *Infect. Immun.,* 77, 5216-5224.

[61] Schaller, M., Korting, H.C., Borelli, C., Hamm, G., and Hube, B. (2005). *Candida albicans*-secreted aspartic proteinases modify the epithelial cytokine response in an *in vitro* model of vaginal candidiasis. *Infect. Immun.,* 73, 2758-2765.

[62] Pietrella, D., Rachini, A., Pandey, N., Schild, L., Netea, M., Bistoni, F., Hube, B., and Vecchiarelli, A. (2010). The Inflammatory response induced by aspartic proteases of *Candida albicans* is independent of proteolytic activity. *Infect. Immun.,* 78, 4754-4762.

[63] Pietrella, D., Pandey, N., Gabrielli, E., Pericolini, E., Perito, S., Kasper, L., Bistoni, F., Cassone, A., Hube, B., and Vecchiarelli, A. (2013). Secreted aspartic proteases of *Candida albicans* activate the NLRP3 inflammasome. *Eur. J. Immunol.,* 43, 679-692.

[64] Tavanti, A., Davidson, A.D., Fordyce, M.J., Gow, N.A., Maiden, M.C., and Odds, F.C. (2005). Population structure and properties of *Candida albicans*, as determined by multilocus sequence typing. *J. Clin. Microbiol.,* 43, 5601-5613.

[65] Whiley, R.A., Cruchley, A.T., Gore, C., and Hagi-Pavli, E. (2012). *Candida albicans* strain-dependent modulation of pro-inflammatory cytokine release by *in vitro* oral and vaginal mucosal models. *Cytokine,* 57, 89-97.

[66] Wu, H., Downs, D., Ghosh, K., Ghosh, A.K., Staib, P., Monod, M., and Tang, J. (2013). *Candida albicans* secreted aspartic proteases 4-6 induce apoptosis of epithelial cells by a novel Trojan horse mechanism. *FASEB J.* in press, fj.12-214353.

[67] Hube, B., and Naglik, J. (2001). *Candida albicans* proteinases: resolving the mystery of a gene family. *Microbiology,* 147, 1997-2005.

[68] Taylor, B.N., Staib, P., Binder, A., Biesemeier, A., Sehnal, M., Rollinghoff, M., Morschhauser, J., and Schroppel, K. (2005). Profile of *Candida albicans*-secreted aspartic proteinase elicited during vaginal infection. *Infect. Immun.,* 73, 1828-1835.

[69] Staib, P., Kretschmar, M., Nichterlein, T., Kohler, G., Michel, S., Hof, H., Hacker, J., and Morschhauser, J. (1999). Host-induced, stage-specific virulence gene activation in *Candida albicans* during infection. *Mol. Microbiol.,* 32, 533-546.

[70] Staib, P., Kretschmar, M., Nichterlein, T., Hof, H., and Morschhauser, J. (2000). Differential activation of a *Candida albicans* virulence gene family during infection. *Proc. Natl. Acad. Sci. USA,* 97, 6102-6107.

[71] Naglik, J.R., Moyes, D., Makwana, J., Kanzaria, P., Tsichlaki, E., Weindl, G., Tappuni, A.R., Rodgers, C.A., Woodman, A.J., Challacombe, S.J., et al. (2008). Quantitative expression of the *Candida albicans* secreted aspartyl proteinase gene family in human oral and vaginal candidiasis. *Microbiology,* 154, 3266-3280.

[72] Taylor, B.N., Fichtenbaum, C., Saavedra, M., Slavinsky, I.J., Swoboda, R., Wozniak, K., Arribas, A., Powderly, W., and Fidel Jr, P.L. (2000). *In vivo* virulence of *Candida albicans* isolates causing mucosal infections in people infected with the human immunodeficiency virus. *J. Infect. Dis.,* 182, 955-959.

[73] Fonzi, W.A., and Irwin, M.Y. (1993). Isogenic strain construction and gene mapping in *Candida albicans*. *Genetics,* 134, 717-728.

[74] Bain, J.M., Stubberfield, C., and Gow, N.A. (2001). Ura-status-dependent adhesion of *Candida albicans* mutants. *FEMS Microbiol. Lett.,* 204, 323-328.

[75] Brand, A., MacCallum, D.M., Brown, A.J., Gow, N.A., and Odds, F.C. (2004). Ectopic expression of *URA3* can influence the virulence phenotypes and proteome of *Candida albicans* but can be overcome by targeted reintegration of *URA3* at the *RPS10* locus. *Eukaryot. Cell,* 3, 900-909.

[76] Cheng, S., Nguyen, M.H., Zhang, Z., Jia, H., Handfield, M., and Clancy, C.J. (2003). Evaluation of the roles of four *Candida albicans* genes in virulence by using gene disruption strains that express *URA3* from the native locus. *Infect. Immun.,* 71, 6101-6103.

[77] Lay, J., Henry, L.K., Clifford, J., Koltin, Y., Bulawa, C.E., and Becker, J.M. (1998). Altered expression of selectable marker *URA3* in gene-disrupted *Candida albicans* strains complicates interpretation of virulence studies. *Infect. Immun.,* 66, 5301-5306.

[78] Dunkel, N., and Morschhauser, J. (2011). Loss of heterozygosity at an unlinked genomic locus is responsible for the phenotype of a *Candida albicans* sap4Delta sap5Delta sap6Delta mutant. *Eukaryot. Cell,* 10, 54-62.

[79] Bruno, V.M., Wang, Z., Marjani, S.L., Euskirchen, G.M., Martin, J., Sherlock, G., and Snyder, M. (2010). Comprehensive annotation of the transcriptome of the human fungal pathogen *Candida albicans* using RNA-seq. *Genome. Res.,* 20, 1451-1458.

[80] Kadosh, D., and Johnson, A.D. (2005). Induction of the *Candida albicans* filamentous growth program by relief of transcriptional repression: a genome-wide analysis. *Mol. Biol. Cell,* 16, 2903-2912.

[81] Yin, Z., Stead, D., Selway, L., Walker, J., Riba-Garcia, I., McLnerney, T., Gaskell, S., Oliver, S.G., Cash, P., and Brown, A.J. (2004). Proteomic response to amino acid starvation in *Candida albicans* and *Saccharomyces cerevisiae*. *Proteomics,* 4, 2425-2436.

[82] Gygi, S.P., Rochon, Y., Franza, B.R., and Aebersold, R. (1999). Correlation between protein and mRNA abundance in yeast. *Mol. Cell Biol.,* 19, 1720-1730.

[83] Kamthan, M., Mukhopadhyay, G., Chakraborty, N., Chakraborty, S., and Datta, A. (2012). Quantitative proteomics and metabolomics approaches to demonstrate N-acetyl-D-glucosamine inducible amino acid deprivation response as morphological switch in *Candida albicans*. *Fungal. Genet. Biol.,* 49, 369-378.

[84] Ene, I.V., Heilmann, C.J., Sorgo, A.G., Walker, L.A., de Koster, C.G., Munro, C.A., Klis, F.M., and Brown, A.J. (2012). Carbon source-induced reprogramming of the cell wall proteome and secretome modulates the adherence and drug resistance of the fungal pathogen *Candida albicans*. *Proteomics*, 12, 3164-3179.

[85] Xu, Y., Wang, Y., Yan, L., Liang, R.M., Dai, B.D., Tang, R.J., Gao, P.H., and Jiang, Y.Y. (2009). Proteomic analysis reveals a synergistic mechanism of fluconazole and berberine against fluconazole-resistant *Candida albicans*: endogenous ROS augmentation. *J. Proteome. Res.,* 8, 5296-5304.

[86] Chaffin, W.L. (2008). *Candida albicans* cell wall proteins. *Microbiol. Mol. Biol. Rev.,* 72, 495-544.

[87] Klis, F.M., de Koster, C.G., and Brul, S. (2011). A mass spectrometric view of the fungal wall proteome. *Future Microbiol.,* 6, 941-951.

[88] Kniemeyer, O., Schmidt, A.D., Vodisch, M., Wartenberg, D., and Brakhage, A.A. (2011). Identification of virulence determinants of the human pathogenic fungi *Aspergillus fumigatus* and *Candida albicans* by proteomics. *Int. J. Med. Microbiol.* ,301, 368-377.

[89] Yates, J.R., Ruse, C.I., and Nakorchevsky, A. (2009). Proteomics by mass spectrometry: approaches, advances, and applications. *Annu. Rev. Biomed. Eng.,* 11, 49-79.

[90] Washburn, M.P., Wolters, D., and Yates, J.R., 3rd (2001). Large-scale analysis of the yeast proteome by multidimensional protein identification technology. *Nat. Biotechnol.,* 19, 242-247.

[91] Motokawa, M., Kobayashi, H., Ishizuka, N., Minakuchi, H., Nakanishi, K., Jinnai, H., Hosoya, K., Ikegami, T., and Tanaka, N. (2002). Monolithic silica columns with various skeleton sizes and through-pore sizes for capillary liquid chromatography. *J. Chromatogr., A,* 961, 53-63.

[92] Miyamoto, K., Hara, T., Kobayashi, H., Morisaka, H., Tokuda, D., Horie, K., Koduki, K., Makino, S., Nunez, O., Yang, C., et al. (2008). High-efficiency liquid chromatographic separation utilizing long monolithic silica capillary columns. *Anal. Chem.,* 80, 8741-8750.

[93] Iwasaki, M., Miwa, S., Ikegami, T., Tomita, M., Tanaka, N., and Ishihama, Y. (2010). One-dimensional capillary liquid chromatographic separation coupled with tandem mass spectrometry unveils the *Escherichia coli* proteome on a microarray scale. *Anal. Chem.,* 82, 2616-2620.

[94] Altelaar, A.F., Frese, C.K., Preisinger, C., Hennrich, M.L., Schram, A.W., Timmers, H.T., Heck, A.J., and Mohammed, S. (2012). Benchmarking stable isotope labeling based quantitative proteomics. *J. Proteomics, in press,* doi: 10.1016/j.jprot.2012.10. 009.

[95] Heilmann, C.J., Sorgo, A.G., Siliakus, A.R., Dekker, H.L., Brul, S., de Koster, C.G., de Koning, L.J., and Klis, F.M. (2011). Hyphal induction in the human fungal pathogen *Candida albicans* reveals a characteristic wall protein profile. *Microbiology,* 157, 2297-2307.

[96] Spellberg, B.J., Ibrahim, A.S., Avanesian, V., Fu, Y., Myers, C., Phan, Q.T., Filler, S.G., Yeaman, M.R., and Edwards, J.E., Jr. (2006). Efficacy of the anti-*Candida* rAls3p-N or rAls1p-N vaccines against disseminated and mucosal candidiasis. *J. Infect. Dis.,* 194, 256-260.

[97] Luo, G., Ibrahim, A.S., Spellberg, B., Nobile, C.J., Mitchell, A.P., and Fu, Y. (2010). *Candida albicans* Hyr1p confers resistance to neutrophil killing and is a potential vaccine target. *J. Infect. Dis.,* 201, 1718-1728.

[98] Aoki, W., Ueda, T., Tatsukami, Y., Kitahara, N., Morisaka, H., Kuroda, K., and Ueda, M. (2013). Time-course proteomic profile of *Candida albicans* during adaptation to a fetal serum. *Pathog. Dis.,* 67, 67-75.

[99] Hernandez, R., Nombela, C., Diez-Orejas, R., and Gil, C. (2004). Two-dimensional reference map of *Candida albicans* hyphal forms. *Proteomics,* 4, 374-382.

[100] Martinez-Gomariz, M., Perumal, P., Mekala, S., Nombela, C., Chaffin, W.L., and Gil, C. (2009). Proteomic analysis of cytoplasmic and surface proteins from yeast cells, hyphae, and biofilms of *Candida albicans*. *Proteomics,* 9, 2230-2252.

[101] Pitarch, A., Sanchez, M., Nombela, C., and Gil, C. (2002). Sequential fractionation and two-dimensional gel analysis unravels the complexity of the dimorphic fungus *Candida albicans* cell wall proteome. *Mol. Cell Proteomics,* 1, 967-982.

In: Candida *albicans*: Symptoms, Causes and Treatment Options ISBN: 978-1-62808-882-3
Editors: Leon A. Dietrich and Tim S. Friedmann

Chapter III

A Drug Delivery Approach for the Treatment of *Candida albicans*

María J. Martín Villena* and Beatriz Clares Naveros*
Pharmacy and Pharmaceutical Technology Department. Faculty of Pharmacy, University of Granada, Campus of Cartuja street s/n, Granada, Spain

Abstract

Infections due to *Candida* species are the most common among fungal infections. Although *Candida albicans* is a yeast normally found as part of the skin microbiota, mouth, intestinal tract and vagina. Certain illnesses, stress, or medications can cause the growth of *Candida* out of control producing infections that range from superficial to systemic level, and potentially life-threatening diseases.

Not surprisingly, superficial candidiasis is a common reason for patient visits to dermatologists. On the other hand, the incidence of invasive *Candida* infections have continued to increase over the last decade within high risk patient groups, as those severely immunocompromised patients infected with HIV or under chemotherapy treatment, solid organ or haematopoietic stem cell transplant recipients, and patients in intensive care units. In this way early diagnosis and prompt initiation of antifungal therapy are essential factors to reduce morbidity and mortality.

This chapter provides preliminary information on risk factor for *Candida* infections and symptoms. In addition, current knowledge about pharmaceutical formulation and drug delivery strategies on treatment of multiple forms of candidiasis is discussed.

1. Introduction

There are over 81 known species of *Candida*, but only about eight are considered pathogenic. Among these, the species *C. albicans* is the most frequently isolated from both

* Email: {mjmv, beatrizclares}@ugr.es.

colonized and infected sites. However, other *Candida* species, including *Candida glabrata* and *Candida parapsilosis*, are currently also significant human pathogens [1]. Indeed, it has been suggested that the incidence of infections caused by non-*C. albicans* species is increasing [2, 3].

C. albicans is a polymorphic species that can grow as yeast cells, pseudohyphae and hyphae [4]. It is often present in small numbers in the skin, mouth, intestinal tract, and vagina. However, certain illnesses, stress, or medications can cause the growth of this opportunistic pathogen out of control producing infections that covers a wide spectrum of diseases varying in severity from asymptomatic colonization to superficial mucosal infections to life-threatening disseminated candidiasis [2]. In fact, *Candida* species have become important nosocomial pathogens. In some hospitals, may cause nearly 10% of nosocomial infections. Moreover, because of *Candida* can be transmitted sexually, the Centers for Disease Control and prevention (CDC) classified as a sexually transmitted disease.

Candida infections involve a very complex interaction between a wide range of host factors and yeast virulence determinants that may be differentially expressed depending on the prevailing environmental conditions. One of the most important virulence factors of *C. albicans* is its ability to adhere to certain human tissues. It is quite likely that *C. albicans* possesses surface molecules which serve as a multipurpose adhesins. These adhesins may mediate the attachment or adhesion of the fungus to a multitude of different biological and inert surfaces [5]. But for example in the case of superficial candidiasis is has been proved that it is highly dependent on cell-mediated immunity. The most obvious example is the predisposition of patients with Acquired Immune Deficiency Syndrome (AIDS) to oral and oesophageal candidiasis and their relative resistance, except in the most advanced stages, to disseminated candidiasis, in marked contrast to their susceptibility to other systemic fungal infections [6].

In this chapter we will focus on risk factor for *Candida* infections, symptoms of the most frequently pathologies and also on the current knowledge about formulation and drug delivery strategies on treatment of these diseases.

2. Mucocutaneous Candidiasis

Any other fungus produces a pathological spectrum in humans as *Candida*. The reason why, most of the infections affect the skin or mucous membranes is due to *Candida* is a facultative anaerobe) [7] and these surfaces are very suitable for their growth. The infection usually occurs when the skin is damaged or there is moisture [8].

Mucocutaneous candidiasis (Table 1) presents a wide variety of clinical manifestations with special characteristics in the distinct stages of life. In childhood, candidal napkin dermatitis around the nappy area is common; in adults, many oral manifestations are associated with the use of dental prostheses, and among young adults candidal balanitis and vulvovaginitis are frequent. This infection is both frequent and often resistant among patients with AIDS. The intertrigo is related to humidity and sometimes to diabetes. Candidal perionyxis and onyxis are not common and require an accurate diagnosis for treatment. Candida allergy is controversial and not universally accepted. However, it should be borne in mind in some cutaneous processes [9]. Due to their high prevalence, we will focus on oropharyngeal, vulvovaginal candidiasis and on candidiasis of the skin.

Table 1. Mucocutaneous candidiasis

Oropharyngeal candidiasis
• Pseudomembranous candidiasis
• Erythematous candidiasis
• Atrophic candidiasis
• Hyperplastic candidiasis
• Median rhomboid glossitis
• Angular cheilitis
Genital candidiasis
• Candidal balanitis
• Vulvovaginitis
Candidiasis of the skin
• Candidal napkin dermatitis
• Intertrigo
• Candidal perionyxis and onyxis
• Candidiasis folliculitis
• Nail candidiasis
• Paroniquia acute
• Candida allergy

2.1. Oropharyngeal Candidiasis

With the increased use of antibiotics and immunosuppressive agents, oropharyngeal candidiasis is becoming more common. This infection is also associated with chemotherapy, organ transplantation and with human immunodeficiency virus infection. Others (patients and pathogen) risk factors that predispose to oropharyngeal candidiasis are cited in Table 2 [10, 11].

The commonest form of oral candidiasis is pseudomembranous candidiasis (thrush) which is characterized by inflammation of the oral mucosa with the formation of superficial, elevated, white plaques resembling milk curds. Ulceration may also develop. Initially the lesions may be localised, but they often spread to cover most of the mouth. The lesions may be asymptomatic or associated with pain, burning or dryness of the mouth, loss of taste and pharyngeal dysphagia, nauseas and vomiting. Gastrointestinal bleeding may occur, especially in thrombocytopenic patients [10].

Another form of oropharyngeal candidiasis is the erythematous type, which frequently develops in patients taking antibiotics or using steroid inhalers and in patients with HIV. Patients present red mucosa with loss of papillae on the tongue and patchy red changes in the palate, although any portion of the oral mucosa can be affected. This type of candidiasis is characterized by sensitive and painful erythematous mucosa with few, if any, white plaques [10].

Atrophic candidiasis, is presented in patients with denture stomatitis, or denture sore mouth. The palatal mucosa in contact with the dentures becomes affected and is chronically erythematous and oedematous. A hyperplastic response may be seen, although patients generally experience no symptoms [10].

Hyperplastic candidiasis due to leukoplakia may represent a precancerous condition that presents as bilateral, elevated, white mucosal lesions on the buccal mucosa, tongue, lips, and bottom of the mouth. *Candida* species are frequently cultured from the mouth of patients with common and speckled oral leukoplakia, although they may not be the cause of the lesions. The presence of these organisms may be superficial, and they are thought to be secondary invaders in the epithelial portion of the lesions. Clinical signs and symptoms range from painless plaquelike white patches to nodular erythroplakic lesions that cause the patient discomfort. Smoking appears to be the main risk factor for development of hyperplastic candidiasis [10]. Median rhomboid glossitis is the term used to describe, a red, flat or raised nodular area which is located near to the centre of the tongue. The affected area is missing its normal coating of finger-like projections called filiform papilla, which normally cover the entire top surface of the tongue [12]. Finally, angular cheilitis is an inflammatory reaction at one or both corners of the mouth which is characterized by painful red fissures. *C. albicans* infection is frequently accompanied by *Staphylococcus aureus* infection. Denture wearers and patients with HIV are predisposed to this type of presentation. Although angular cheilitis usually does not indicate a serious disease, severe infections may occur in immunocompromised individuals [10].

Table 2. Risk factors for the development of oropharyngeal candidiasis

Risk factors for development of oropharyngeal candidiasis	
Host factors	Pathogen factors
Age • Neonates • Advanced age Diseases • Diabetes, • Disruption of oral mucosa • Cancer • HIV infection • Malignancies • Xerostomia Drugs • Use of broad-spectrum antibiotics • Steroids • Cancer therapy Dietary factors • High-carbohydrate Diet • Iron-deficiency anaemia Others • Wearing of dentures • Smoking	• Adhesins • Germ tube formation • Presence of mycelia • Production of endotoxins • Induction of tumour necrosis factor • Production of acid proteinase • Phenotypic switching

Candida infections of the mouth and throat must be treated with prescription antifungal medication since untreated infections can lead to a more serious form of invasive candidiasis. Normally, oral candidiasis responds to topical treatments such as clotrimazole troches and nystatin suspension (nystatin swish and swallow). Clotrimazole troches are more palatable than nystatin oral suspension and may be used in patients who cannot tolerate the taste of nystatin [13]. It should also be taken into account that the combination of nystatin with chlorhexidine digluconate, resulting in the treatment failure [14, 15].

Oesophageal candidiasis is typically treated with oral fluconazole or itraconazole. For severe or azole-resistant oesophageal candidiasis, treatment with amphotericin B may be necessary. Systemic agents have to be used when topical therapy has been ineffective or not tolerated, primarily in immunocompromised (intravenous).

2.1.1. Topical Dosage Forms

As we indicate before, for the treatment of this infection, topical preparations should always be used before systemic antifungal drugs because they are not absorbed systemically [16]. Topical drugs avoid the systemic adverse effects and drug interactions of the systemic agents. These topical agents are available in an assortment of pharmaceutical formulations, including oral rinses, troches, powder, and creams [10].

The selected medication should reflect the conditions in the oral cavity, the severity of the infection and patient-specific factors such as age and immune status. Such factors as taste and texture, and whether sucrose or alcohol is a component of the medication should be considered when selecting a medication and formulation too. On the one hand, many of the oral products include high concentrations of sucrose and thus have a high cariogenic potential, which is particularly important in dentate patients with dry mouth. On the other hand, in patients with dry mouth, tablets given to dissolve in the mouth may be poorly soluble and present a rough surface to the oral soft tissue that could become irritating; oral suspensions may be a good choice for such patients. Cream forms of appropriate medications may be readily applied to the tissue surface of dentures, but their taste and texture may not be tolerated if they are applied without an occlusive appliance [10]. Another disadvantage of this dosage form is that salivary action may dilute and rapidly eliminate topical drugs from the oral cavity, thus rendering them ineffective [17]. Therefore, a mucoadhesive sustained release formulation could be advantageous compared to commonly use of conventional pharmaceutical dosage forms.

2.1.1.1. Mucoadhesive Dosage Forms

Bioadhesive dosage forms can reduce the dosage frequency as they are able to produce a sustained release of the antifungal drug while remaining adhered to the mucosa surface. Among novel mucoadhesive drug delivery systems, tablets and films are the most prominent. Llabot et al. [18] designed a mucoadhesive tablets containing nystatin, in which swellable polymers were responsible for bioadhesion and release modulation. However, buccal films offer advantages over adhesive tablets in terms of flexibility and comfort. Buccal films are also suitable for protecting wound surfaces, which is important when the affection produces ulcerative lesions [19].

2.1.1.2. Nanoemulsions

Fernández et al. [20] suggested that high and sustained nystatin levels in mouth are not a determinant factor for the improvement of the treatment efficacy because nystatin shows a marked postantifungal effect. Owing to this fact, other pharmaceutical forms, different from mucoadhesive systems, can be used to tackle effectively oral candidosis, solving the oral suspension problems. In this sense, Nanoemulsions which are transparent (translucent) dispersions of two immiscible phases, with a mean droplet size in the nanometric scale (from 20 to 200 nm) can be used. They have been reported to be stable formulations against sedimentation or creaming, and they are well known systems that enhance the solubility of lipophilic drugs. From the pharmaceutical point of view, nanoemulsions possess improved transdermal and dermal delivery properties *in vitro* and *in vivo* over classical dosage forms. The adequate selection of the nanoemulsion components allows the development of formulations with harmless effect on the buccal mucosa contrary to mucoadhesive buccal devices.

2.1.2. Systemic Dosage Forms

Systemic agents have been used when topical therapy has been ineffective or not tolerated, primarily in immunocompromised or in patients with *Candida* esophagitis.

2.1.2.1. Oral Dosage Forms

The trouble is that some of the drugs used for the oral treatment of candidiasis have low aqueous solubility which produces low bioavailability in oral administration. This is the case of azoles. But, if dissolution rates and apparent solubility is increased, the bioability of these drugs can be enhanced solving the problem [21]. Some strategies have been developed to improve this aspect, as for example: i) formation of drug/cyclodextrin complexes, [22, 23] ii) solubilisation in surfactant systems (Self-emulsifying drug delivery systems) [24, 25] and iii) solid-state manipulation, which implies the dispersion of the drug particles into a solid matrix [26].

2.1.2.2. Injectable Dosage Forms

The high hydrophobicity of azole antifungals has to be taken into account in the development of injectables too. For this reason an intravenous liposomal formulation of itraconazole has been designed to modify the pharmacokinetics and enhance concentrations at the site of infection [27]. Itraconazole (Sporanox® I.V., manufactured by Janssen Pharmaceutica Products, L.P.) has also been solubilised by complexation with hydroxypropyl-β-cyclodextrin (HPBCD). However, the toxicity and side effects caused by the vehicle limit its application. As an alternative, itraconazole nanosuspensions were produced by high pressure homogenization of aqueous suspensions by the company Baxter applying their so-called NANOEDGE™ technology. In comparative studies with Sporanox® I.V., the nanosuspension composition containing itraconazole demonstrated good tolerability and efficacy *in vivo* [28]. Similarly, Rabinow et al. [29] reported an intravenous itraconazole nanosuspension produced by a tandem process of microcrystallization followed by homogenization. This new formulation demonstrated that itraconazole nanosuspension formulations may enhance their antifungal efficacy with improved tolerability.

Table 3. Recommendation for the treatment of oropharyngeal candidiasis

Class and Agent	Oropharyngeal
Polyenes	
• Nystatin	Primary(Mild illness)
• Amphotericin B	Alternative(refractory illness)
Imidazoles	
• Clotrimazole	Primary (Mild illness)
• Miconazole	
• Ketoconazole	
• Butoconazole	
• Tioconazole	
• sertaconazole	
Triazole	
• Fluconazole	Primary (severe-moderate illness)
• Itraconazole	Alternative(refractory illness)
• Voriconazole	Alternative(refractory illness)
• Posaconazole	Alternative(refractory illness)
• Econazole	Alternative(refractory illness)
• Terconazole	
Echinocadins	Alternative(refractory illness)
• Caspofungin	
• Anidolafungin	
• Micafungin	
Others	Wearing of dentures
• Chlorhexidine gluconate 0,2%	
• Denture cleanser	

An itraconazole nanocrystal formulation (NCF) has also been prepared by NanoCrystal® technology, which involves milling larger crystals of itraconazole in the surfactant poloxamer 338 [30]. The itraconazole NCF may therefore provide an alternative to Sporanox® I.V. solution, with potentially less toxicity by omitting ciclodextrines in the formulation.

Itraconazole injectable emulsions have been reported too. These are made by solubilisation by emulsification technique, or referred to as SolEmuls® technology [28]. Since itraconazole is poorly soluble in both aqueous and oily phases of the emulsion, incorporation is only possible by localizing the drug in the lecithin bilayer at the oil-water interface by homogenization. Nanocapsules, a nanometric colloidal carrier that possesses an oily core surrounded by a polymeric wall with lipophilic and/or hydrophilic surfactants at the interface have also been applied to azoles due to the ability of nanocapsules to modify the biopharmaceutical properties of lipophilic substances.

It should be also pointed out, that the use of nanocapsules containing technetium-99m labelled fluconazole, may be a suitable and promising intravenous formulation to identify infectious foci and treat disseminated candidiasis [31]. However, *in vivo* studies are required for further investigation.

2.2. Vulvovaginal Candidiasis

Other mucocutaneus infections caused by *C. albicans* are vulvovaginal candidiasis (VVC). VVC is the most common cause of infectious vaginitis, representing between 40% and 50% of all of cases. An estimated 75% of women will have at least one episode of VVC, and 40–45% will have two or more episodes [32]. Some risk factors for yeast infection are HIV positive, diabetes, recent use of antibiotics.

Typical symptoms of VVC include pruritus, vaginal soreness, dyspareunia, external dysuria, and discomfort during urination, infertility, reduction of the sexual pleasure and abnormal vaginal discharge. VVC is classified as complicated or uncomplicated based on frequency, symptoms, microbiology and response to treatment. VC complicated appears in 10–20% of women and is much more difficult to treat.

2.2.1. Treatment of Vulvovaginal Candidiasis

To treat uncomplicated VVC, short-course topical formulations (i.e., single dose and regimens of 1–3 days) are effective (Table 4). Treatment with azoles results in relief of symptoms and negative cultures in 80–90% of patients who complete therapy. The creams and suppositories in this regimen are oil-based and might weaken latex condoms and diaphragms.

Complicated VVC includes cases of severe VVC, VVC caused by non-*C. albicans* species, VVC associated with pregnancy and recurrent VVC (RVVC) and immunocompetent women such as HIV-infected women.

Table 4. Recommendation for the treatment of vulvovaginal candidiasis

Class and Agent	Uncomplicated VVC	Complicated VVC
Polyenes • Nystatin	X	
Imidazoles • Clotrimazole • Miconazole • Butoconazole • Tioconazole	X	Alternative in RVVC
Triazole • Fluconazole	X (A single dose)	RVVC (a dose per week for 6 months) after control of the episode with a topical or oral azole
Others • Flucystosine • Boric acid		Non-albicans species In combination with amphotericin B

2.2.1.1. Recurrent Vulvovaginal Candidiasis

RVVC, usually defined as four or more episodes of symptomatic VVC in 1 year, affects a small percentage of women (<5%). The pathogenesis of RVVC is poorly understood, and most women with RVVC have no apparent predisposing or underlying conditions. Vaginal cultures should be obtained from patients with RVVC to confirm the clinical diagnosis and to identify unusual species (including non-albicans *Candida* species).

Each individual episode of RVVC caused by *C. albicans* responds well to short-duration oral or topical azole therapy.

However, to maintain clinical and mycologic control, some specialists recommend a longer duration of initial therapy to attempt mycologic remission before initiating a maintenance antifungal regimen.

The first line therapy is oral fluconazole (i.e., 100 mg, 150 mg, or 200 mg dose) weekly for 6 months. If this regimen is not feasible, topical treatments used intermittently as a maintenance regimen can be considered. Suppressive maintenance antifungal therapies are effective in reducing RVVC. However, 30–50% of women will have recurrent disease after maintenance therapy is discontinued [32].

2.2.1.2. Severe Vulvovaginal Candidiasis

Severe vulvovaginitis (i.e., extensive vulvar erythema, oedema, excoriation, and fissure formation) is associated with lower clinical response rates in patients treated with short courses of topical or oral therapy. Either 7–14 days of topical azole or 150 mg of fluconazole in two sequential doses (second dose 72 hours after initial dose) is recommended [32].

2.2.1.3. Pregnancy

VVC frequently occurs during pregnancy. Only topical azole therapies, applied for 7 days, are recommended for use among pregnant women [32].

2.2.1.4. HIV Infection

Vaginal *Candida* colonization rates among HIV-infected women are higher than among those for seronegative women. Therapy for VVC in HIV-infected women should not differ from that for seronegative women. Although long-term prophylactic therapy with fluconazole at a dose of 200 mg weekly has been effective in reducing *C. albicans* colonization and symptomatic VVC, this regimen is not recommended for routine primary prophylaxis in HIV-infected women in the absence of recurrent VVC [32].

2.2.2. New Treatments of Vulvovaginosis

Despite the availability of effective antimicotic treatments, the high recurrence rate of local vaginal infections shows that the management of these prevalent conditions needs to be improved. With this objective novel pharmaceutical formulations have been designed. These systems should provide a long retention time to maximize drug release, a proper spreading over the vaginal epithelium to obtain fast absorption or to maximize the effect in case of local treatment and has also to be easy to administer and not cause discomfort to improve patient compliance.

2.2.2.1. Bioadhesive Effervescent Tablets

Bioadhesive effervescent tablets containing ketoconazole have been reported for vaginal delivery to overcome gastrointestinal disturbances such as nausea and vomiting associated with orally administered formulations. The results show sustained release properties [33].

2.2.2.2. Mucoadhesive Vaginal Creams

Mucoadhesive vaginal creams of itraconazole have been tested. These creams retained vaginally in a rabbit model and human clinical studies, apart from being safe and well tolerated [34]. Furthermore, they were highly effective in reducing or eliminating fungal cultures with few adverse effects due to non-systemic absorption. Similarly, addition of a bioadhesive polymer to econazole nitrate vaginal ovules led to a greater frequency of negative culture and reduced recurrence rate after applying for 3 days to women with vaginal candidiasis [35].

2.2.2.3. Solid Lipid Nanoparticles and Nanostructured Lipid Carriers

Another reported strategy, has been the design of solid lipid nanoparticles (SLN) and nanostructured lipid carriers (NLC) which are colloidal carrier systems composed of physiological and biodegradable lipids of low toxicity [36]. Both SLN and NLC possess a number of features advantageous for topical application, including protection of labile drugs against chemical degradation, controlled release of the drug, prolonged residence time of formulation in the stratum corneum and targeting of drug to the upper layers of the skin [37]. They were also reported to have occlusive properties as a result of barrier film formation after application [38].

2.2.2.4. Liposomes and Niosomes

The apparent increase in biophasic availability brought about by the incorporation of active principle into liposomal delivery and release systems has led to an interest in their development and possible therapeutic applications [39]. The use of topical liposomes has been shown to enhance the penetration of vesicle-bound drugs into the skin and act as drug localizers, with low systemic absorption and sustained drug release locally. Niosomes, an analogous to liposomes, are closed bilayer structures of self-assembled non-ionic amphiphiles in aqueous media. They have higher chemical stability, intrinsic skin penetration-enhancing properties and a lower cost compared to liposomes [40].

Liposomal and niosomal clotrimazole incorporated into a carbopol gel for vaginal administration has been reported [41]. The results demonstrated prolonged and enhanced antifungal activity of the liposomal and niosomal formulations, relative to a control drug containing gel and a marketed clotrimazole ointment.

Additionally, the liposome and niosome gels were well tolerated. This study suggested alternative formulations for clotrimazole and other antifungal azoles could provide sustained and controlled release of drug for local vaginal therapy. Topical application of niosomes behaves similar to liposomes *in vivo*, with a prolonged contact time of drug with the applied tissues, thus illustrating the potential of drug in niosomes to improve skin penetration and accumulation in the superficial skin strata.

2.2.2.5. Microparticles

Microparticles can be useful instead of traditional dosage forms since allow controlling the drug release, reducing number of doses required, protect the drug from inactivation and reduce the drug toxicity. Martín-Villena et al. [42] developed a formulation of nystatin loaded microcapsules by complex coacervation coated with polymeric surfactants chitosan and poloxamer 407. The results showed the ability of these systems to adhere to the vaginal mucosa. Moreover nystatin loaded microparticles exhibited a clear inhibition effect on the *C. albicans* growth, and specially chitosan coated microparticles suggesting their clinical potential use, once assured the security of the treatment by the permeation studies performed.

2.2.2.6. Probiotics

The administration of probiotics may have a role in the treatment of VVC, through restoration of the normal vaginal microbiota. But probiotics are not only useful for the treatment of vulvovaginal candidiasis but it can also be used for bacterial vaginitis and oral candidiasis. These microorganisms produce a low vaginal pH through fermentation of lactose and glycogen to lactic acid, which is a strong producer of hydrogen peroxide. Probiotics also display competitive adherence with pathogens to epithelial cells, since some of them can produce biosurfactants, which discourage the growth of pathogens by inhibiting adhesion of microorganisms along cells [43].

Moreover, probiotics may co-aggregate with pathogens to block the adhesion and /or displace previously adherent pathogens on vaginal epithelial [44]

In this sense, the identification of the adhesins with which *Candida* adhere to the host cells will also serve as markers for invasive diseases or as vaccine components to boost waning local mucosal immunity as in recurrent candidal vaginitis. Or perhaps, helping to interrupt the adherence of *Candida* to the host cell may serve as adjunctive therapy to antifungals or probiotic in some forms of the disease [5].

2.3. Candidal Skin Infections and Paronychia

Candidiasis of the skin is often confined to body folds, including the interdigital spaces of hands or feet. Typically, small satellite pustules lie distal to the periphery of the rim of rash. Paronychia (nail-fold infections) can be also caused by *Candida*.

2.3.1. Candidiasis Folliculitis

They are rare and occur in brown heroine consumers. It is a septicaemia which is accompanied by painful pustules on the scalp and face. The infection of the retina is frequent with risk of blindness [45].

2.3.2. Intertrigo

Intertrigo refers to inflammation of opposed skin and commonly occurs in the inframammary region, axillae, groin, gluteal folds, and between redundant skin folds of the abdominal pannus in obese patients. Intertrigo is thought to be caused by friction between skin folds which, when combined with heat and moisture, leads to maceration and inflammation. Intertrigo is a common condition, and patients considered most at risk for intertrigo include those with poor hygiene, diabetes, or obesity [46].

2.3.3. Candidal Napkin Dermatitis

Diaper dermatitis is the most common cutaneous disorder of infancy and early childhood. The list of culpable factors of this dermatitis includes mechanical friction, moisture and increase in skin hydration, contact with urine and faeces and their degradation products (which can cause irritation as well as increased skin permeability to other irritants), faecal proteolytic and lipolytic digestive enzymes, variations in skin pH, superinfection with bacteria and *Candida* species, and other factors.

Candida albicans frequently contaminates diaper dermatitis and should be considered present in any diaper dermatitis known to have persisted for longer than 3 days [47].

2.3.4. Candidal Perionyxis and Onyxis

These infections are common on the hands and are due to the presence of *C. albicans*, but *C. parapsilosis* and *C. guilliermondii*, can also be involved. Onyxis often occurs after a perionyxis, but it can be primitive and start at the free edge of the nail [45].

2.3.5. Treatment of Candidal Skin Infections and Paronychia

Treatment of *Candida* infections involves topical azoles or polyene antifungals. Oral fluconazole or itraconazole may be necessary in more severe infections and in immunocompromised patients.

Firstly, in the case of intertrigo, candidal perionyxis, candidal onyxis and candidal napkin dermatitis, it is necessary the protection from humidity and maceration of the area [45]. For the intertrigo, the application of an azole, ciclopiroxolamine, amphotericin B or sertaconazole in the form of a lotion, cream or gel for at least 15 days is also required. Some intertrigo, especially in paediatric and elder patient, can extend to great areas of the skin requiring a longer course of treatment.

In candidal onyxis, the nail has to be removed and a filmogenic agent has to be applied. For the treatment of perionyxis a cream with imidizole has to be applied each day. To treat candidal napkin dermatitis join to the administration of a topical azole can be used hydrocortisone, and it is recommend covering the cream with a second layer of a paste.

Finally, a nystatin nanoemulsion for skin application has been recently reported with good *in vitro* results [48].

3. Systemic Candidal Infection

Candidemia describes the presence of *Candida* species in the blood. It occurs only in individuals who are severely ill and/or immunocompromised. Systemic infections are frequently associated with patients with neutropenia, for example as a result of antineoplastic therapy or immunosuppressive therapy associated with organ transplantation, those with indwelling intravascular lines, and those receiving antibiotics or parenteral nutrition are at risk for *Candida* septicaemia too.

3.1. Treatment of Systemic Infection

All forms of systemic disease are serious, progressive, and potentially deadly. When a treatment is chosen it should be kept in mind the physiological state of the patient (neutropenic or non-neutropenic) and previous treatments (Table 5).

The increased incidence of systemic mycoses caused by *Candida* species in hospitalized patients is an important cause of morbidity and mortality worldwide, especially in critically ill patients. Biofilms play an important role in the perpetuation of these infections primarily with respect to their ability to adhere to various medical devices and tissues. Biofilms are biological communities with a high degree of organization, in which microorganisms form structured, coordinated and functional communities. These biological communities are embedded in a self-created extracellular matrix. Moreover, biofilm production is associated with a high level of antimicrobial resistance of the associated organisms. The ability of *Candida* species to form drug-resistant biofilms is an important factor in their contribution to human disease [49].

The study of plants such as *Arnica montana, Artemisia absinthium* and *Urtica dioica*, have attracted great attention [50]. These extracts have shown to present antimicrobial activity against planktonic fungal and bacterial growth; as well as an effect on formation and development of biofilm was shown in *S. aureus* and *C. albicans*.

Another promising antifungal strategy is the use of silver nanoparticles (AgNPs). Silver is a well-known antimicrobial agent and has a long history of application in medicine with a well-tolerated tissue response and a low toxicity profile.

Table 5. Recommended treatment for candidemia

Class and Agent	Candidemia Nonneutropenic adults	Candidemia Neutropenic patients
Polyenes • Amphotericin B	Alternative	Primary
Imidazoles • Clotrimazole • Miconazole • Ketoconazole • Butoconazole • Tioconazole • sertaconazole	Primary (Mild illness)	
Triazole • Fluconazole • Voriconazole	Primary Alternative	Alternative Alternative
Echinocadins • Caspofungin • Anidolafungin • Micafungin	Primary (Moderately severe to severe illness and in patients with recent azole exposure)	Primary

The use of AgNPs has been suggested for coating medical titanium implants [51–53] in the hope of inhibiting biofilm formation and thereby reducing the incidence of microbial infections and rejection. Silver has been shown to interfere with microbial DNA replication within bacteria and fungi. It makes these particles a desirable and promising antifungal effect, with no serious side effects to the host.

Furthermore, anti-*Candida* antibodies can reduce the binding of *Candida* to various surfaces [54, 55]. Studies with antibodies have been performed by various authors to test their effects on various fungal and bacterial organisms. IgY inhibited *C. albicans* biofilm formation. This anti-*C. albicans* IgY may have a protective effect against oral candidiasis and reduce the dissemination of *Candida* species.

Therefore, anti-*C. albicans* IgY could be considered for prophylactic immunotherapy under limited conditions [56].

More recently, the application of photodynamic therapy has been investigated regarding its inactivation of micro-organisms that are pathogenic to the human host. Several authors have associated light emitting diodes (LEDs) with other substances [57–59].

3.3. Treatment: Systemic Infection in Paediatric Patients

The prevention and treatment of infection in paediatric patients is still limited by the facts that not all antifungal agents are approved for paediatrics, the appropriate dosage of these drugs has not been established for all age groups, and postmarketing data providing information on the safety and efficacy of approved agents under real-life circumstances are scant [60].

Options as a first-line therapy for invasive candidiasis approved by the Food and Drug Administration (FDA) and/or the European Medicines Agency (EMA) for all paediatric age groups includes liposomal amphotericin B, fluconazole, caspofungin and micafungin [61–64]. Criteria for selecting the initial treatment include the clinical status of the patient, organ impairment, concomitant medications, pretreatment with antifungal agents, the *Candida* species isolated and its resistance pattern.

Candidiasis can also appear after childbirth. Congenital candidiasis is characterized by a variety of clinical features ranging from a diffuse erythematous skin eruption, with or without vesicles and pustules, to systemic disease in which the lungs are usually affected and can also be associated with intrauterine or neonatal death due to disease dissemination [65].

For these reasons, congenital candidiasis should be considered in the differential diagnosis of neonatal generalized maculopapular or pustular skin eruptions, along with; some other disorders such as *Listeria monocytogenes* infection, impetigo, chickenpox, herpes virus infection, syphilis and epidermolysis bullosa may appear. Infants with systemic fungal infections (i.e., positive blood, urine and/or CSF cultures) commonly present respiratory distress and an elevated white blood cell count with a left shift, reaching the level of a leukemoid reaction, particularly within the first 3 days of life. Persistent hyperglycemia and glycosuria have also been reported [66]. It has been recognized, that in fullterm infants with congenital candidiasis and skin involvement alone, the clinical course is often benign, and only topical therapy or no therapy at all is required. In infants with respiratory distress and clinical and laboratory signs of sepsis however, systemic antifungal therapy with amphotericin B is recommended [67]. Wang et al. [65] indicated the presence of characteristic skin lesions caused by *Candida* species, occurring within 24 hours of birth could help in the early diagnosis of congenital candidal infection. This early recognition and treatment could increase the chance of a favourable outcome.

Additionally, it has to be taken into account that the treatment of invasive candidiasis in pregnant women, most of the azoles, including fluconazole, itraconazole, and posaconazole, should generally be avoided because of the possibility of birth defects associated with their use (C category). There are fewer data concerning the echinocandins, but these should be used with caution during pregnancy (C category). Flucytosine and voriconazole are contraindicated during pregnancy because of foetal abnormalities observed in animals (D category). For these reasons the treatment of choice will be systemic amphotericin B [68].

Conclusion

Antifungal potency and drug bioavailability at the site of infection are key factors in determining the therapeutic efficacy of an antifungal agent in the treatment of candidiasis. It is important, since the low concentration of drug at the infection sites may induce antifungal resistance.

For these reasons, there is a need for an effective control of fungal infections, with less toxic formulations, and better patient compliance. In this sense, novel drug delivery systems and therapies are developing. Some of the factors that are essential to be enhanced are: i) the physical and chemical properties of the drugs, ii) delivery of therapeutically relevant doses at the site of infection, iii) as well as a reduction of the systemic toxicities associated with these drugs and the excipients used in some pharmaceutical formulations.

To sum up, the advances drugs formulations and therapies discussed in this chapter are promising. However, many of these data are limited to *in vitro* or animal studies. Further work is needed to translate these findings into the clinical data in order to benefit patients at risk for or suffering from candidiasis.

References

[1] Matthews, R. & Burnie, J. (1998). The epidemiology and pathogenesis of candidiasis: applications in prevention and treatment. *Bulletin de l'Institut Pasteur*, 96, 249–256.

[2] Hoepelmana, I.M. & Dupont, B. (1996). Oral candidiasis: the clinical challenge of resistance and management. *International Journal of Antimicrobial Agents,* 6, 155–159.

[3] Sangeorzan, J.A., Bradley, S.F., He, X., Zarins, L.T., Ridenour, G.L., Tiballi, R.N. et al. (1994). Epidemiology or oral candidiasis in HIV-infected patients: colonization, infection, treatment, and emergence of fluconazole resistance. *American Journal Medicine,* 97, 339–346.

[4] Sullivan, D.J., Moran, G.P., le Pinjon, E., Al-Mosaid, A., Stokes, C., Vaughan, C. et al. (2004). Comparison of the epidemiology, drug resistance mechanisms, and virulence of *Candida dubliniensis* and *Candida albicans*. *FEMS Yeast Research*, 4, 369–376.

[5] Pendrak, M.L. & Klotz, S.A. (1995). Adherence of *Candida albicans* to host cells. *FEMS Microbiology Letters,* 129, 103–114.

[6] Matthews, R., Burnie, J., Smith, D., Clark. I., Midgley J., Conolly, M. et al. (1988). Candida and AIDS: evidence for protective antibody. *Lancet,* 2, 236–266.

[7] Dumitru, R., Hornby, J.M. & Nickerson. K.W. (2004). Defined anaerobic growth medium for studying *Candida albicans* basic biology and resistance to eight antifungal drugs. *Antimicroial Agents Chemotherapy,*48, 2350–2354.

[8] Prescott, L.M., Harley, J.P. & Klein, D.A. (2004). Microbiologia (5ed). Madrid, Spain: McGrawHill.

[9] Rodríguez-Pichardo, A. & García-Bravo, B. (2006). Candidiasis cutaneomucosas. Manifestaciones clínicas. *Medicina Clínica,* 126, 20–24.

[10] Epstein, J.B. & Polsky, B. (1998). Oropharyngeal candidiasis: a review of its clinical spectrum and current therapies. *Clinical Therapeutics,* 20, 40–57.

[11] Peterson, D.E. (1992). Oral candidiasis. *Clinics in Geriatric Medicine*, 8, 513–527.

[12] Van der Wal, N. & Van der Waal, I. (1986). *Candida albicans* in median rhomboid glossitis. *International Journal of Oral and Maxillofacial Surgery*, 15, 322–325.

[13] Owens N.J., Nightingale, C.H., Schweizer, R.T., Schauer, P.K., Dekker, P.T. & Quintiliani, R. (1984). Prophylaxis of oral candidiasis with clotrimazole troches. *Archives of Internal Medicine,* 144, 290–293.

[14] Barkvoll, P. & Attramadal, A. (1989). Effect of nystatin and chlorhexidine digluconate on *Candida albicans. Oral Surgery, Oral Medicine, Oral Pathology, and Endodontology,* 67, 279–81.

[15] Barkvoll, P. & Hurlen, B. (1989). Conventional treatment of oral candidiasis-New aspects. *Den Norske tannlaegeforenings tidende, 99*, 116–1 19.

[16] Epstein JB. Oral and pharyngeal candidiasis. (1989). *Postgraduate Medical Journal,* 85,257–269.

[17] Samaranayake L.P. & Ferguson M.M. (1994). Delivery of antifungal agents to the oral cavity. *Advanced Drug Delivery Reviews*, 13, 161–179.

[18] Llabot, J.M., Manzo, R.H. & Allemandi, D.A. (2004). Drug release from carbomer: carbomer sodium salt matrices with potential use as mucoadhesive drug delivery system. *International Journal Pharmamaceutics,* 276, 59–66.

[19] Llabot, J.M., Palma, S.D., Manzo, R.H. & Allemandi, D.A. (2007). Design of novel antifungal mucoadhesive films Part I. Pre-formulation studies. *International Journal of Pharmaceutics,* 330, 54–60.

[20] Fernández Campos, F., Calpena Campmany, A.C., Rodriguez Delgado, G., López Serrano, O. & Clares Naveros, B. (2012). Development and characterization of a novel nystatin-loaded nanoemulsion for the buccal treatment of candidosis: ultrastructural effects and release studies. *Journal of Pharmaceutical Sciences*, 101, 3739–3752.

[21] Yang, W., Wiederhold, N.P. & Williams, R.O. (2008). Drug delivery strategies for improved azole antifungal action. *Expert Opinion on Drug Delivery,* 5, 1199–1216.

[22] Loftsson, T. & Brewster, M.E. (1996). Pharmaceuticalapplications of cyclodextrins .1. Drug solubilization and stabilization. *Journal of Pharmaceutical Sciences,* 85, 1017–1025.

[23] Brewster, M.E., Vandecruys, R., Verreck, G. & Peeters, J. (2008). Supersaturating drug delivery systems: effect of hydrophilic cyclodextrins and other excipients on the formation and stabilization of supersaturated drug solutions. *Pharmazie,* 63, 217–220.

[24] Hong, J.Y., Kim, J.K., Song, Y.K., Park, J.S. & Kim, C.K. (2006). A new self-emulsifying formulation of itraconazole with improved dissolution and oral absorption. *Journal of Control Release,* 110, 332 –338.

[25] Woo, J.S., Song, Y.K., Hong, J.Y. & Kim C.K. (2008). Reduced food-effect and enhanced bioavailability of a self-microemulsifying formulation of itraconazole in healthy volunteers. *European Journal of Pharmaceutical Sciences*, 33, 159–65.

[26] Kapsi, S.G. & Ayres, J.W. (2001). Processing factors in development of solid solution formulation of itraconazole for enhancement of drug dissolution and bioavailability. *International Journal of Pharmamaceutics*, 229, 193–203.

[27] Leconte, P., Joly, V., Saintjulien, L., Gillardin, J.M., Carbon, C. & Yeni, P. (1992). Tissue distribution and antifungal effect of liposomal itraconazole in experimental cryptococcosis and pulmonary aspergillosis. *American Review of Respiratory Diseases*, 145, 424–429.

[28] Akkar A. & Muller, R.H. (2003).Intravenous itraconazole emulsions produced by SolEmuls technology. *European Journal of Pharmaceutics and Biopharmaceutics,* 56, 29–36.

[29] Rabinow, B., Kipp, J., Papadopoulos, P., Wong, J., Glosson, J., Gass, J., et al. (2007). Itraconazole IV nanosuspension enhances efficacy through altered pharmacokinetics in the rat. *International Journal of Pharmaceutics,* 339, 251–260.

[30] Mouton, J.W., van Peer, A., de Beule, K., Van Vliet, A., Donnelly, J.P. & Soons, P.A. (2006). Pharmacokinetics of itraconazole and hydroxyitraconazole in healthy subjects after single and multiple doses of a novel formulation. *Antimicrobial Agents and Chemotherapy,* 50, 4096–4102.

[31] de Assis, D.N., Mosqueira, V.C., Vilela, J.M., Andrade, M.S. & Cardoso, V.N. (2008). Release profiles and morphological characterization by atomic force microscopy and photon correlation spectroscopy of (99m) Technetium-fluconazole nanocapsules. *International Journal of Pharmaceutics,* 349, 152–60.

[32] Workowski, K.A. & Berman, S. (2010). Sexually transmitted diseases treatment guidelines. *Centers for Disease Control and Prevention, MMWR*, 59 (No. RR-12), 1–110.

[33] Wang, L. & Tang, X. (2008). A novel ketoconazole bioadhesive effervescent tablet for vaginal delivery: design, in vitro and 'in vivo' evaluation. *International Journal of Pharmaceutics,* 350, 181–187.

[34] Francois, M., Snoeckx, E., Putteman, P., Wouters, F., De Proost, E.D., Delaet, U., et al. (2003). A mucoadhesive, cyclodextrin-based vaginal cream formulation of itraconazole. *AAPS Pharmsci Journal,* 5, 50–54.

[35] Furneri, P.M., Corsello, S. & Masellis, G. (2008). Econazole-polycarbophil, a new delivery system for topical therapy: microbiological and clinical results on vaginal candidiasis. *Journal of Chemotherapy,* 20, 336–340.

[36] Muller, R.H., Mader, K. & Gohla, S. (2000). Solid lipid nanoparticles (SLN) for controlled drug delivery – a review of the state of the art. *European Journal of Pharmaceutics and Biopharmaceutics,* 50, 161–177.

[37] Souto, E.B., Wissing, S.A., Barbosa, C.M. & Muller, R.H. (2004).Development of a controlled release formulation based on SLN and NLC for topical clotrimazole delivery. *International Journal of Pharmaceutics,* 278, 71–77.

[38] Wissing S.A., Lippacher, A. & Muller, R.H. (2001). Investigations on the occlusive properties of solid lipid nanoparticles (SLN). *Journal of Cosmetic Science,* 52, 313–324.

[39] Clares, B., Gallardo, V., Medina, M.M., & Ruiz, M.A. (2009). Multilamellar liposomes of triamcinolone acetonide: preparation, stability, and characterization. *Journal of Liposomal Research*, 19, 197–206.

[40] Ning, M.Y., Guo, Y.Z., Pan, H.Z., Chen, X. & Gu, Z. (2005). Preparation, in vitro and in vivo evaluation of liposomal/niosomal gel delivery systems for clotrimazole. *Drug Development and Industrial Pharmacy,* 31, 375 –83.

[41] Yuen, C. W. M., Yip, J., Liu, L., Cheuk, K., Kan, C. W., Cheung, H. C. & Cheng, S.Y. (2012). Chitosan microcapsules loaded with either miconazole nitrate or clotrimazole, prepared via emulsion technique. *Carbohydrate Polymers,* 89, 795–801.

[42] Martín-Villena, M.J., Fernández-Campos, F., Calpena-Campmany, A.C., Bozal-de Febrer, N., Ruiz-Martínez, M.A. & Clares-Naveros, B. (2013). Novel microparticulate systems for the vaginal delivery of nystatin: Development and characterization *Carbohydrate Polymers,* 94, 1– 11.

[43] Valraeds M.M., van der Mei HC, Reid, G. & Busscher, H.J. (1996).Inhibition of initial adhesion of uropathogen Enterococcus faecalis by biosurfactants from Lactobacillus isolates. *Applied and Environmental Microbiology,* 62, 1958–1963.

[44] Barrons, R., & Tassone, D. (2008). Use of *Lactobacillus* probiotics for bacterial genitourinary infection in women: A review. *Clinical Therapeutics, 30*, 453-468.

[45] Contet-Audonneau, N. & Schmutz, J.L. (2001). Antifongiques et mycoses superficielles. *Revue Française des Laboratoires,* 332, 37–48.

[46] Collier, C. (2007). Within the fold: Treatments of intertrigo. *Journal of the American Academy of Dermatology*, 56, AB126.

[47] Jain, A., Jain, S. & Rawat, S. (2010). Emerging fungal infections among children: A review on its clinical manifestations, diagnosis, and prevention. *Journal of Pharmacy and Bioallied Sciences*, 2, 314–320.

[48] Fernandez-Campos, F., Clares Naveros, B., López Serrano, O., Alonso Merino, C. & Calpena Campmany, A.C. (2013). Evaluation of novel nystatin nanoemulsion for skin candidosis infections. *Mycoses,* 56, 70–81.

[49] Sardi, J.C., Scorzoni, L., Bernardi, T., Fusco-Almeida, A.M. & Mendes Giannini, M.J. (2013).Candida species: current epidemiology, pathogenicity, biofilm formation, natural antifungal products and new therapeutic options. *Journal of Medical Microbiology*, 62, 10–24.

[50] Stanciuc, A.M., Gaspar, A., Moldovan, L., Saviuc, C., Popa, M. & Marutescu, L. (2011). In vitro antimicrobial activity of Romanian medicinal plants hydroalcoholic extracts on planktonic and adhered cells. *Roumanian Archives of Microbiology and Immunology,* 70, 11–14.

[51] Huang, T., Cao, W., Elsayed-Ali, H.E. & Xu, X.H. (2012). High-throughput ultrasensitive characterization of chemical, structural and plasmonic properties of EBL-fabricated single silver nanoparticles. *Nanoscale,* 4, 380–385.

[52] Lu, X.O., Zhang, B.L., Wang, Y.B., Zhou, X.L., Weng, J., Qu, S.X., et al. (2011). Nano-Ag-loaded hydroxyapatite coatings on titanium surfaces by electrochemical deposition. *Journal of the Royal Society Interface,* 8, 529–539.

[53] García-Contreras, R., Argueta-Figueroa, L., Mejía-Rubalcava, C., Jiménez-Martínez, R., Cuevas-Guajardo, S., Sánchez-Reyna, P.A., et al. (2011). Perspectives for the use of silver nanoparticles in dental practice. *International Dental Journal,* 61, 297–301.

[54] López-Ribot, J.L., Casanova, M., Murgui, A. & Martínez, J.P. (2004). Antibody response to Candida albicans cell wall antigens. *FEMS Immunology & Medical Microbiology,* 41, 187–196.

[55] Bujdáková, H., Paulovicová, E., Borecká-Melkusová, S., Gasperík, J., Kucharíková, S., Kolecka, A., et al. (2008). Antibody response to the 45 kDa *Candida albicans* antigen in an animal model and potential role of the antigen in adherence. *Journal of Medical Microbiology,* 57, 1466–1472.

[56] Fujibayashi, T., Nakamura, M., Tominaga, A., Satoh, N., Kawarai, T., Narisawa, N., et al. (2009). Effects of IgY against Candida albicans and Candida spp. adherence and biofilm formation. *Japanese Journal of Infectious Diseases.* 62, 337–342.

[57] Chen, C.P., Chen, C.T. & Tsai, T. (2012). Chitosan nanoparticles for antimicrobial photodynamic inactivation: characterization and in vitro investigation. *Photochemistry and Photobiology,* 88, 570–576.

[58] Junqueira, J.C., Jorge, A.O., Barbosa, J.O., Rossoni, R.D., Vilela, S.F., Costa, A.C., et al. (2012). Photodynamic inactivation of biofilms formed by Candida spp., Trichosporon mucoides, and Kodamaea ohmeri by cationic nanoemulsion of zinc 2,9,16,23-tetrakis(phenylthio)- 29H, 31H-phthalocyanine (ZnPc). *Lasers in Medical Science,* 27, 1205–1212.

[59] Ribeiro, A.P., Andrade, M.C., da Silva Jde, F., Jorge, J.H., Primo, F.L., Tedesco, A.C., et al. (2012). Photodynamic inactivation of planktonic cultures and biofilms of *Candida albicans* mediated by aluminum-chloride-phthalocyanine entrapped in nanoemulsions. *Photochemistry and Photobiology,* 89, 111−119

[60] Groll, A.H. (2011). Efficacy and safety of antifungals in pediatric patients. *Early Human Development* 87, 71–74.

[61] Zaoutis, T.E, Jafri, H.S., Huang, L.M., Locatelli, F., Barzilai, A., Ebell, W., et al. (2009). A prospective, multicenter study of caspofungin for the treatment of documented Candida or Aspergillus infections in pediatric patients. *Pediatrics,* 123, 877–884.

[62] Maertens, J.A., Madero, L., Reilly, A.F., Lehrnbecher, T., Groll, A.H., Jafri, H.S., et al. (2010). A randomized, double-blind, multicenter study of caspofungin versus liposomal amphotericin B for empiric antifungal therapy in pediatric patients with persistent fever and neutropenia. *Pediatric Infectious Disease Journal,* 29, 415–420.

[63] Groll, A.H. & Tragiannidis, A. (2010). Update on antifungal agents for pediatric patients. *Clinical Microbiology Infection,* 16, 1343–1353.

[64] Groll, A.H. & Tragiannidis, A. (2009). Recent advances in antifungal prevention and treatment. *Seminars in Hematology,* 46, 212–229.

[65] Wang, S.M., Hsu, C.H. & Chang, J.H. (2008). Congenital Candidiasis. *Pediatrics and Neonatology,* 49, 94−96.

[66] Pradeepkumar, V.K., Rajadurai, V.S. & Tan, K.W. (1998). Congenital candidiasis: varied presentations. *Journal of Perinatology,* 18, 311−316.

[67] Darmstadt, G.L., Dinulos, J.G. & Miller, Z. (2000). Congenital cutaneous candidiasis: clinical presentation, pathogenesis, and management guidelines. P*ediatrics,* 105, 438−444.

[68] Moudgal, V.V. & Sobel, J.D. (2003). Antifungal drugs in pregnancy: a review. Expert *Opinion Drug Safety,* 2, 475–483.

In: Candida *albicans*: Symptoms, Causes and Treatment Options ISBN: 978-1-62808-882-3
Editors: Leon A. Dietrich and Tim S. Friedmann

Chapter IV

Proteins and Peptides as Potential Antifungals for Treating *Candida albicans* Infections

Tzi Bun Ng*, Jack Ho Wong* and Charlene Cheuk Wing Ng
School of Biomedical Sciences, Faculty of Medicine,
The Chinese University of Hong Kong,
New Territories, Hong Kong, China

Abstract

A multitude of peptides and proteins including lactoferrin, the lactoferrin-derived peptides lactoferrampin and lactoferricin and their chimera, and other lactoferrin-derived peptides ; human, mammalian and submammalian defensins and cathelicidins , salivary histatin 5 and salivary glycoproteins, IQ-motif peptides, human thrombin C-terminal peptides, lysozyme, calprotectin, serum amyloid A, interleukin-2 and lipopolysaccharides have been found to be potential anti-Candida therapeutic agents.Their inhibitory actions on *Candida albicans* are reviewed.

Keywords: *Candida albicans,* lactoferrin, lactoferrampin, lactoferricin, defensins, cathelicidins, salivary histatin 5, lysozyme, interleukin-2, lipopolysaccharides

Introduction

In view of the emergence of resistance of *Candida albicans* to existing drugs, a search for new drugs is warranted. Antimicrobial peptides and proteins have been proposed to be

* Emails of corresponding authors: b021770@mailserv.cuhk.edu.hk (TBNg), jack1993@yahoo.com (JHWong), fax: 852 26035123, phone: 852 39436872.

promising agents for treatment of infections caused by *Candida albicans.* A diversity of such peptides and proteins with therapeutic potential is discussed in the following.

Lactoferrin (LF) is an iron-binding glycoprotein found in milk and various external secretions. It manifests a host of activities encompassing antimicrobial, anti-cancer, antioxidant, and immunomodulatory effects (Ye et al., 2011).

Defensins are cationic antimicrobial peptides produced for defense against assault of pathogens by a diversity of organisms as phylogenetically remote as mammals, subnannalian vertebrates, invertebrates, plants and fungi. Alpha-defensins were first found in mammalian neutrophils. Beta-defensins were discovered in mammalian neutrophils and epithelia and also in avian leukocytes. Theta-defensins found in monkeys are cyclic structures formed by the ligation of two truncated alpha-defensins (Antcheva et al., 2006). Mammalian defensins exert an antimicrobial action and regulate innate and adaptive immunity (Antcheva et al., 2006). The counterparts of mammalian defensins have been detected and/or isolated from an array of plant and submammalian animal species and a sizeable amount of information has accumulated.

The term 'cathelicidins' was proposed in 1995 by Zanetti and his colleagues to refer to the C-terminal peptides that manifest antimicrobial activity following cleavage from cathelin. They possess a cathelin-like sequence as well as a cationic antimicrobial domain. The name takes into account the evolutionary relationship of the novel protein family to cathelin (Zanetti et al., 1995). Contemporary evidence indicates that cathelicidins may play a role in host defense, causing the pathogen to succumb by direct inactivation as well as by other means.

Human Lactoferrin (Lf)

Viability test and electron microscopy revealed that the growth inhibitory effect of human milk mediated by lactoferrin on *C. albicans*is was fungistatic rather than fungicidal (Andersson et al. 2000).

The candidacidal action of human lactoferrin was impeded by K(+) and Na(+) concentrations exceeding 30 mM and by (Ca(2+) and Mg(2+) in excess of 4 mM. Cellular release of K(+), cytosolic acidification, and an alteration in membrane potential seen in lactoferrin-treated *C. albicans* cells signified interaction of lactoferrin with the cytoplasmic membrane. Changes in metabolic state induced by anerobic conditions and mitochondrial inhibitors such as azide, antimycin, carbonyl cyanide m-chlorophenylhydrazone, and 2, 4-dinitrophenol undermined the candidacidal activity of lactoferrin (Viejo-Díaz e al., 2004).

Neonatal Wistar rats were infected subcutaneously with *C. albicans, S. epidermidis* or both, at doses of 200 million colony-forming units.The rats were randomly allocated into three groups. The groups received intraperitoneal administrations of recombinant human lactoferrin at 40 mg/kg/day or 300 mg/kg/day, or saline, once daily for 4 days. It was found that lactoferrin prophylaxis significantly improved survival in the coinfected group at 40 mg/kg/dose (by 16.1%) and at 300 mg/kg/dose (by 15.1%;) and in the *S. epidermidis* group at a dose of 40 mg/kg/dose (by 18.6%). Survival in coinfected and in the *S. epidermidis* infected group (40 mg/kg/dose) was enhanced through indirect mechanisms (Venkatesh et al., 2007).

Lactoferrin exerted broad- spectrum antimicrobial activity against pathogenic *C. albicans, E. coli,* and *Staphylococcus aureus* in the digestive tract of a transgenic milk-fed animal model and protected small intestinal mucosa from damage (Yen et al., 2011).

Recombinant Human Lactoferrin

Recombinant human lactoferrin acted synergistically with commonly used anti-Candida drugs (amphotericin B and fluconazole) and appears to be a promising therapeutic agent that awaits clinical evaluation (Venkatesh and Rong 2008).

Production of Human Lactoferrin in Animal Milk

Transgenic mice were bred by employing genetic constructs carrying the human lactoferrin gene which were produced as a result of the concerted efforts of Russian and Belorussian scientists. The maximum human lactoferrin concentration in the milk was 160 g/L.Transgenic goats were also produced and up to 10 g human lactoferrin was found in a liter of their milk. Experimental goatherds that produced hLf in their milk were also bred, and recombinant hLf was identical to the natural lactoferrin in physicochemical properties and fungicidal activity against *C. albicans* (Goldman et al. 2012).

Tissue Conditioner Capable of Binding with Human Lactoferrin

Tissue conditioner containing cation exchange resin bound human lactoferrin and exerted an anti-microbial action against *C. albicans*. The physical properties of the tissue conditioner, which were harmless to human fibroblasts, were satisfactory. The tissue conditioner is expected to increase the local concentration of lactoferrin in saliva at the lesion site and hence may be useful for the prevention and treatment of denture stomatitis and systemic opportunistic infections (Yamamoto et al., 2009).

Bovine Lactoferrin

The growth inhibitory action of human neutrophils on *C. albicans* escalated in the presence of human Lf at concentrations which alone had no inhibitory effects. Comparable results were obtained when bovine Lf or iron-saturated bovine Lf , but not human transferrin, was added to human or murine neutrophils. The minimum inhibitory concentration (MIC) of antifungal azoles including clotrimazole, fluconazole, ketoconazole, and itraconazole was lowered by 25% to 6.25% in the presence of a sub-MIC level of bovine Lf, peptic hydrolysate of bovine Lf, or bovine lactoferricin. Other antifungals, such as amphotericin B, nystatin, and flucytosine did not demonstrate synergism with these Lf-related molecules. The anti-Candida activity of bovine Lf or bovine lactoferricin in combination with clotrimazole was shown to be synergistic.Compared with azole-susceptible strains, clinically isolated azole-resistant *C.*

albicans strains were more susceptible to bovine Lf or bovine lactoferricin. Growth of an azole-resistant strain in the presence of fluconazole declined after exposure to sub-MIC levels of bovine Lf or bovine lactoferricin. The data indicate that Lf-related molecules may exert an antifungal action in conjunction with neutrophils and thus modulate azole antifungal effectiveness *in vivo* (Wakabayashi et al., 1998).

Porcine Lactoferrin

Partial degradation of LF by pepsin can give rise to peptides termed lactoferricin (LFcin) with more potent antimicrobial activity. LF and LFcin have been shown to inhibit the growth of a number of pathogenic bacteria (including E. coli and antibiotic-resistant strains), fungi, and even viruses in both in vitro and in vivo studies. We previously demonstrated that both recombinant porcine LF (pLF) produced from yeast and a synthetic 20-residue porcine LFcin peptide exhibit antimicrobial activity in vitro. In one of our recent studies, we performed pathogen challenges, including pathogenic E. coli, Staphylococcus aureus and Candida albicans, of the digestive tract of a transgenic milk-fed animal model.The results showed that LF has broad spectrum antimicrobial activity in the digestive tract and protects the mucosa of the small intestine from injury. Our following study also revealed that pLF as a feedstuff additive enhances avian immunity, including antibody formation and cell-mediated immunity. All of these results suggest that LF could be a novel natural protein in the treatment and prevention of infections with E. coli or antibiotic-resistant bacteria strains (Yen et al., 2011).

Bovine Lactoferricin

Lactoferricin B derived from acid-pepsin digestion of bovine lactoferrin was bactericidal against *C. albicans* and a wide range of bacteria. Lactoferricin probably exerts a transient antimicrobial effect at mucosal surfaces (Jones et al., 1994).Bovine lactoferricin showed antimicrobial activity against *C. albicans, C. tropicalis* and *C. neoformans* (Vorland et al; 1998). The concentrations of lactoferrin, its pepsin hydrolysate or bovine lactoferricin required to inhibit the growth of *C. albicans* were reduced in the presence of relatively low concentrations of clotrimazole, but not when polyene and fluoropyrimidine antifungal agents were present. The minimum inhibitory concentration (MIC) of the antifungal azoles tested was reduced by 6.25%-25% in the presence of a sub-MIC level of lactoferrin, its pepsin hydrolysate or bovine lactoferricin (Wakabayashi et al., 1996).

Synthetic Bovine Lactoferricin

The 20-residue porcine lactoferricin displayed antimicrobial activity against *Escherichia coli* ATCC25922, *Staphylococcus aureus* ATCC25923, and *Candida albicans* ATCC14053. The minimal inhibitory concentrations and minimal bactericidal concentrations of porcine lactoferricin ranged from 12 to 25 microM when tested in bacteria and fungi. Porcine lactoferricin was 4 times more efficacious than human lactoferricin, but had an only slightly attenuated effectiveness compared with bovine lactoferricin (Chen et al., 2006).

Lactoferricin, Lactoferrampin and Chimera

Lactoferricin and lactoferrampin are two antimicrobial peptides found in the N-terminal lobe of bovine lactoferrin with broad-spectrum antimicrobial activity against *C. albicans*. A heterodimer designated as LFchimera, in which lactoferrampin and lactoferricin were joined at their C-terminals through the two amino groups of a single Lys residue, has elevated antimicrobial activity compared to lactoferrampin and lactoferricin or an equimolar mixture of the two peptides. Differential scanning calorimetry studies demonstrated that lactoferrampin, lactoferricin and LFchimera all affected the thermotropic phase behavior of anionic phospholipid suspensions. Calcein leakage and vesicle fusion experiments using anionic liposomes disclosed that LFchimera had more potent membrane perturbing activity compared to lactoferrampin and lactoferricin.

The NMR solution structure unveiled that the helical content in LFchimera rose compared to lactoferricin and lactoferrampin due to the Lys linkage, but the relative orientations of lactoferricin and lactoferrampin with respect to each other were not fixed (Haney et al., 2012).

Antimicrobial Peptide from the Lactoferrampin-Domain of Bovine Lactoferrin

A 32-mer fragment obtained from the endoproteinase AspN digestion of bovine lactoferrin demonstrated potent antimicrobial activity. Desalted crude digest exhibited higher antimicrobial activity than native bovine lactoferrin (Bolscher et al., 2006).

LFampin 265-284

Amino acid residues essential to the anti-Candida albicans activity of LFampin 265-284 derived from bovine lactoferrin were identified by a glycine substitution scan. Each single replacement of a cationic amino acid ensued in a marked decrement in candidacidal activity, for each residue to a different extent. Substitution within the helix-facilitating N-terminal sequence DLIW produced a less drastic consequence, for instance, the activity was somewhat attenuated after replacement of Ile and Trp (van der Kraan et al., 2005).

Human Lactoferrin –Derived Peptide hLF1-11

hLF1-11 displayed anti- *Candida albicans* activity *in vitro* and forestalled infections with fluconazole-resistant *Candida albicans* in animal experiments. Since hLF1-11 is inactive *in vitro* at physiological salt concentrations, van der Does et al. (2010) suggested modulation of the immune system as an additional mechanism of action of the peptide. Brief treatment of monocytes with hLF1-11 during GM-CSF-induced differentiation brought about differentiation of monocytes to a macrophage subset with both pro- and anti-inflammatory cytokine production, heightened responsiveness to microbial structures and high efficacy against *C. albicans* (van der Does et al., 2010).

Synthetic Human Lactoferrin -Derived Peptides HL9 and HLopt2

Starting from the N-terminal end, downsizing of peptide sequence 14-31 from the N-terminal end, corresponding to the antibacterial alpha-helix of human lactoferrin (LF), showed that the peptide sequence 19-31 (KCFQWQRNMRKVR, HL9) was the optimal length for antimicrobial activity.

Alanine scanning of peptide sequence 20-31 showed that Cys20, Trp23, Arg28, Lys29, or Arg31 was important for expressing full killing activity, particularly against *C. albicans*. Substituting the neutral hydrophilic amino acids Gln24 and Asn26 for Lys and Ala (HLopt2), respectively, enhanced microbicidal activity significantly against all test organisms compared to the amino acids natural counterpart, also, in comparison with HL9, HLopt2 had more than 10-fold-stronger fungicidal activity. Furthermore, HLopt2 was less affected by metallic salts than HL9. The microbicidal activity of HLopt2 was slightly reduced only at pH 7.0, as tested in the pH range of 4.5 to 7.5. The results showed that the microbicidal activity of synthetic peptide sequences, based on the antimicrobial alpha-helix region of LF, can be significantly enhanced by optimizing the length and substitution of neutral amino acids at specific positions, thus suggesting a sequence lead with therapeutic potential (Håversen et al., 2010).

HLopt2, a modified peptide sequence (CFQWKRAMRKVR) based on the N-terminal amino acid residues 20-31 of human lactoferrin (hLF), killed *Candida albicans, Candida kefyr, Candida krusei, Candida parapsilosis,* and *Cryptococcus neoformans,* at in vitro concentrations of 12.5-25 μg/mL, but not *Candida glabrata*. HLopt2 had over 16-fold higher killing activity than a double-sized human lactoferricin-like peptide HLBD1 (amino acid residues 16-40). By inducing some helical formation caused by lactam bridges or by extending the assay time (from 2h to 20 h), HLBD1 became almost comparable with HLopt2 in its fungicidal activity. Killing of *C. albicans* cells by HLopt2 was rapid and was accompanied by cytoplasmic and mitochondrial membrane permeabilisation as well as formation of deep pits on the yeast cell surface. In a murine *C. albicans* skin infection model, atopic treatment with the peptides resulted in significantly reduced yields of Candida from the infected skin areas.The antifungal activities of HLopt2 in vitro and in vivo suggest possible potential as a therapeutic agent against most Candida spp. and C. neoformans. The greatly improved antifungal effect of the lactam-modified HLBD1 indicates the importance of amphipathic helix formation for lethal activity Kondori et al., 2011.

Human Lactoferrin -Derived Peptides, Lfpep and kaliocin-1

The synthetic peptide Lfpep, a cationic peptide with bactericidal and giardicidal activities, possesses the sequence from positions 18 to 40 of human lactoferrin. The synthetic peptide kaliocin-1 is a novel bactericidal peptide that possess the sequence from positions 153 to 183 of human lactoferrin. Both peptides were active against Candida spp., including fluconazole- and amphotericin B-resistant clinical isolates. Lfpep exhibited 8- to 30-fold higher antifungal activity and increased salt resistance compared with kaliocin-1. Lfpep but not kaliocin-1 permeabilized the membrane of *Candida albicans* cells. The amino acid sequence of kaliocin-1 contains the "multidimensional antimicrobial signature" which is conserved in disulfide-containing antimicrobial peptides and manifests high homology to brevinin-1Sa, a frog skin antimicrobial peptide (Viejo-Díaz et al., 2005). These features may be of interest in the design of new antifungals.

Human β-Defensins

One, two and three disulfide bridges have been introduced into the peptides corresponding to the N-terminal segments of HBD4. Augmented antimicrobial activity resulted when there were three disulfide bridges. The antimicrobial potency was analogous to that of HBD4 and was reduced in the presence of salt. The peptides gain entry into fungal cells quickly without permeabilizing the membrane and exert their action within the cells and not at the membrane (Sharma and Nagaraj, 2012).

Reduced Human β-Defensin 1

Human β-defensin 1 (hBD-1) with the disulfide bridges reduced has a high inhibitory potency against *C. albicans*. Reduced hBD-1 is structurally different from oxidized hBD-1 and free cysteines at the C-terminal are important for the bactericidal effect.The thioredoxin (TRX) system reduces hBD-1 *in vitro* and TRX is found together with reduced hBD-1 in human epithelia. Reduced hBD-1 protects the healthy epithelium from colonisation by opportunistic fungi and commensal bacteria (Schroeder et al., 2011).

Human β-Defensin 3 (DEFB103)

Purified human β-defensin 3 (DEFB103) demonstrated strong antimicrobial activities against *C. albicans* (Dong et al., 2011).Recombinant human β-defensin 3rHBD3 exhibits antibacterial activity against oral pathogenic strains that adhere to maxillofacial silicone elastomer, and may, thus, contribute to the prevention of infections caused by *C. albicans* and *S. aureus* (Shi et al., 2009).

Rhesus Macaque Oral Alpha- Defensin

The synthetic peptide ROAD-1 corresponding to fully processed rhesus macaque oral alpha-defensin exhibited concentration-dependent inhibition of *C. albicans*. It adopts the canonical disulfide pairing and alpha-defensin fold although it has unique surface features. It is known that the antimicrobial mechanism of defensins correlates with the ability to disrupt and permeabilize the cell envelope which in turn depends on the surface features of the folded peptide (Vasudevan et al., 2008).

Rhesus Macaque Theta Defensins

The three rhesus macaque theta defensins (RTD 1-3) and protegrin 1 (PG-1) manifested analogous antimicrobial activity against *C. albicans* in 10 mM buffers at pH 7.4. Physiologic sodium chloride concentrations reduced the antimicrobial activity of the RTDs. RTDs were neither cytotoxic nor hemolytic, in contrast to PG-1. The low cytotoxicity of the RTDs did not depend on the peptides' cyclic conformation (Tran et al., 2008).

Recombinant Mouse β- Defensin 3

Recombinant mouse β-defensin 3 inhibited *C. albicans* growth (MIC, 25 μg/ml), and demonstrated fungicidal activity against *C. albicans* (MFC, 100 μg/ml). Cells treated with rMBD3 displayed morphological and ultrastructural alterations, encompassing delamination and perforation of peripheral cell walls, porosity, and inanition of cytoplasmic contents. rMBD3 exhibited synergy with itraconazole, amphotericin or 5-fluorocytosine in their actions against the two C. albicans strains tested (Jiang et al., 2012).

Peroxisome Proliferator-Activated Receptor Gamma

Peroxisome proliferator-activated receptor gamma (PPARgamma) maintains constitutive expression of beta-defensin in the colon, DEFB1 in humans and mDefB10 in mice. Colonic mucosa of Ppargamma mutant animals could not effectively kill intestinal *C. albicans, Bacteroides fragilis, Enterococcus faecalis,* and *Escherichia coli.* A functional promoter variant required for DEFB1 expression protects against Crohn's colitis and ileocolitis. The results advocate the development of PPARgamma-targeting therapeutic and/or nutritional strategies to suppress colonic inflammation by reinstating antimicrobial immunity (Peyrin-Biroulet et al., 2010).

Synthetic Antimicrobial Decapeptide KSL-W

KSL-W was devoid of toxicity on cell adhesion or growth, indicating its safety when used on human cells. KSL-W impaired the adhesion and growth of *Candida albicans* on engineered human oral mucosa epithelium. The subsequent expression of Toll-like receptors and human β-defensins in tissues infected with KSL-W-treated Candida was diminished. KSL-W and the antifungal drug amphotericin B regulated secretion of the proinflammatory cytokine IL-1β and IL-6 by the epithelial cells in an analogous way. Hence the virulence of KSL-W Candida is reduced by KSL-W via modulation of host innate immunity (Semlali et al., 2011).

Defensin -NV from the Venom of the Ectoparasite Wasp

Nasonia Vitripennis

Defensin-NV, with 52 amino acids and 3 disulfide bridges and the sequence VTCELLMFGGVVGDSACAANCLSMGKAGGSCNGGLCDCRKTTFKELWDKRFG, exhibits homology to other insect defensins, was highly potent against fungi Gram-positive bacteria, and Gram-negative bacteria (Ye et al., 2010).

Crotamine from the Venom of Crotalus Durissus Terrificus

Crotamine is a highly basic nonhemolytic β-defensin peptide from the venom of *Crotalus durissus terrificu* with potent antifungal activity against *Candida* spp., *Cryptococcus neoformans* and *Trichosporon* spp. It induced marked ultrastructural changes in *C. albicans* but has low cytotoxicity toward nontumormammal cell lines (HEK293, PC12, and primary culture astrocyte cells) (Yamane et al., 2013).

Purple Pole Bean Defensin

A pH-stable and thermostable defensin from *Phaseolus vulgaris* cv. 'Extra-long Purple Pole inhibited mycelial growth in *Candida albicans* with a potency (IC50 4.8 microM) higher than that of the plant defensin coccinin (IC50>50 microM). It induced SYTOX Green uptake and thus membrane permeabilization in C. albicans, but had no effect erythrocyte membrane permeability (Lin et al., 2009).

Human Cathelicidin (LL-37) and Mouse Cathelicidin (mCRAMP)

The human cathelicidin LL-37, and mouse cathelicidin mCRAMP appear active against *C. albicans*, but may be most effective as a superficial barrier to infection (López-García et al., 2005).

Mammalian Cathelicidins

The cathelicidins SMAP29 and CAP18 manifested an inhibitory action against oral bacteria and clinically important oral yeasts including *C. albicans, C. krusei, C. tropicalis, Actinobacillus actinomycetemcomitans, Fusobacterium nucleatum, Porphyromonas gingivalis,* and *Streptococcus sanguis* (Guthmiller et al., 2001). Some organisms (*C. albicans,* methicillin-resistant *S. aureus,* and *Proteus mirabilis*) were susceptible in low-salt media but were resistant to LL-37 in media that contained 100 mM NaCl (Turner et al., 1998).

Guinea Pig Cathelicidin

Guinea pig cathelicidin CAP11 (G1-I43) possesses potent antimicrobial activities. The active antibacterial domain resides at G1 to R18 of CAP11. The hydrophilicity (positive charge) of the peptide (1-18m2) was increased by replacing G1 with K and Q14 with R. 1-18m2 possesses a therapeutic potential for *C. albicans* and bacterial infections (Okuda et al., 2009).

Salivary Histatin 5

Non-immune salivary proteins comprising histatins, lactoferrin, lactoperoxidase, and lysozyme, contribute to innate host defense in the oral cavity. Salivary histatin 5 destroys *C. albicans* by binding to membrane proteins and non-lytic release of cellular ATP. Extracellular ATP may then activate fungal ATP receptors to bring about cell death (Edgerton and Koshlukova, 2000).

Surface coating acrylic with chlorhexidine or histatins 5 suppressed *C. albicans* biofilm growth and has potential therapeutic application (Pusateri et al., 2009).

Defensins, Protegrins, Histatins and Lactoferrin –Derived Peptides

Analogs of antimicrobial peptides such as defensins, histatins, lactoferrin-derived peptides and protegrins, and combinations of these peptides with antifungal drugs, have been tested for the therapy of candidiasis (Lupetti et al., 2002).

Salivary Glycoproteins

The suppression of *C. albicans* adhesion to oral epithelial cells by saliva is dependent on mannose residues on salivary glycoproteins.Mannose is a binding ligand on *C. albicans* and epithelial cells. Anticancer therapy reduces salivation and the concentrations of salivary glycoproteins inhibiting *C. albicans* adhesion and hence induce oral C. albicans overgrowth (Umazume et al., 1995).

IQ-Motif Peptides

The IQ-motif is an amphipathic, often positively charged, α-helical, calmodulin binding sequence found in a number of eukaryote signalling, transport and cytoskeletal proteins. They have biophysical characteristics amalogous to those of α-helical cationic antimicrobial peptides like human cathelicidin LL-37. Some peptides with the sequences of IQ-motifs derived from the human cytoskeletal scaffolding proteins IQGAP2 and IQGAP3 displayed inhibitory activity against *C. albicans* and low haemolytic activity (McLean et al., 2013).

Human Thrombin C-Terminal Peptides

A peptide variant, GKYGFYTHVFRLKKWIQKVI (G Y20), of the C-terminal region of human thrombin exhibits low toxicity and a preserved antimicrobial as well as anti-inflammatory effect, showed efficiency in mouse models of LPS shock and P. aeruginosa sepsis. The work defines structure-activity relationships of C-terminal host defense peptides of thrombin and delineates a strategy for selecting peptide epitopes of therapeutic interest Kasetty et al., 2011.

Lysozyme

The exposure of both *C. albicans* and *C. tropicalis* isolates to an azole (fluconazole) and two polyene drugs (amphotericin B, nystatin) enhanced fungal susceptibility to lysozyme but not to lactoferrin. Exposure to the two polyene drugs had a lesser impact on the lysozyme susceptibility of both Candida species compared with the azole drug. *C. tropicalis* was more susceptible than *C. albicans* to lysozyme (Anil et al., 2002).

Antimicrobial Factors in the Cervial Mucus Plug

The cervical mucus plug is located between the vagina which has an abundance of microorganisms and the uterine cavity which is normally sterile, indicating a host defense function. Cervical mucus plugs collected from healthy women at parturition and the aqueous plug extracts demonstrated antifungal activity against *C albicans*. Lactoferrin, lysozyme, neutrophil defensins, and secretory leukoprotease inhibitor were found in the extracts at levels high enough to exert antimicrobial activity (Hein et al., 2002).

Calprotectin from Rat Peritoneal Exudate Cells

The growth inhibition of *C. albicans* by murine neutrophils was augmented by the addition of a low concentration of the antimicrobial protein calprotectin. In conjunction with calprotectin, lactoferrin potently suppressed the growth of *C. albicans* (Okutomi et al., 1998).

Serum Amyloid A

Serum amyloid A is a 12-kDa protein secreted in bulk quantities by hepatic cells during microbial infections or inflammatory diseases. It induces chemotaxis of PMN, monocytes, and T lymphocytes and enhances the adhesion of these cells to endothelial monolayers. The recombinant protein, at levels similar to serum concentrations observed during an acute phase response, strongly activates PMN leading to a fast and transient rise of cytosolic calcium level and increase of cell-surface expression of antigens like CD11c and CD16 which are implicated in adhesion and microbial recognition. Concomitantly there is an augmented lactoferrin secretion and anti-Candida activity. Thus serum amyloid A may be part of a potential host antifungal defense mechanism (Badolato et al., 2000).

Interleukin-2 (IL-2)

Freshly isolated human PMN constitutively express detectable surface levels of IL-2R beta as well as mRNA for IL-2R beta. The rapid and dose-dependent IL-2 enhancement of antifungal activity against *C. albicans* could be prevented by an antiserum against IL-2R beta or antilactoferrin antibodies. PMN release of lactoferrin but not superoxide anion production accounted for the heightened activity against *C. albicans* in IL-2-treated PMN 9 (Djeu et al., 1993).

Lipopolysaccharides

Lipopolysaccharides (LPSs) from *Escherichia coli, Serratia marcescens,* and *Salmonella typhimurium*, at doses from 1 to 100 ng/ml, strongly enhanced growth inhibition of *C. albicans* by human PMN *in vitro*. Flow cytometry analysis disclosed that LPS markedly augmented phagocytosis of *C. albicans* cells by increasing the number of yeasts ingested per neutrophil as well as the number of neutrophils capable of ingesting fungal cells. LPS activation stimulated release of lactoferrin. Lactoferrin antibodies undermined the anti-*C. albicans* activity of both LPS-stimulated and unstimulated PMN. Northern blot analysis revealed elevated generation of mRNAs of interleukin-1 beta, interleukin-6 and tumor necrosis factor alpha, and in neutrophils within 1 h of LPS stimulation. The data show that bacterial LPSs boost neutrophil function against *C. albicans* and that the lactoferrin released may account for the antifungal effect of PMN. PMN play an extraphagocytic, immunomodulatory role during infection (Palma et al., 1992).

Mannoprotein Fraction of *Candida Albicans*

One mannoprotein fraction of *C. albicans,* MP-F2, potentiated PMN inhibition on growth of yeast and mycelial forms of *C. albicans in vitro,* as potently as bacterial lipopolysaccharide, granulocyte-macrophage colony-stimulating factor, and interleukin-8, by increasing the actual number of phagocytic PMN and augmenting the release of lactoferrin which exhibited an anti-candidal action without PMN. The aforementioned observations were reversed by anti-lactoferrin antibodies (Palma et al., 1992).

Conclusion

The different peptides and proteins and lipopolysaccharides referred to above are all capable of inhibiting the growth of *C. albicans.*In some cases the peptides and proteins have been shown to be nontoxic to normal cells and lacking in hemolytic activity which are desirable characteristics. Efficacy *in vivo* has also been demonstrated for some of the peptides and proteins using animal models of infection with *C. albicans*.However, the anti-Candida mechanism awaits elucidation in many cases.As time goes on, it is anticipated that the mechanisms will be unraveled and the structures of some of the aforementioned peptides and proteins can be modified to reduce their toxicity and improve their efficacy for clinical application.

Acknowledgments

The award of a research fund for the control of infectious diseases (grant number 10090812) from Food and Health Bureau, the Government of Hong Kong, is gratefully acknowledged.

References

Andersson Y, Lindquist S, Lagerqvist C, Hernell O. Lactoferrin is responsible for the fungistatic effect of human milk. *Early Hum. Dev.* 2000;59(2):95-105.

Anil S, Samaranayake LP. Impact of lysozyme and lactoferrin on oral Candida isolates exposed to polyene antimycotics and fluconazole. *Oral Dis.* 2002;8(4):199-206.

Antcheva N, Zelezetsky I, Tossi A. Cationic antimicrobial peptides-the defensins. In: Handbook of Biologically Active Peptides (Kastin AJ ed.) 2006; Chapter 11, pp.55-66. Elsevier Inc.

Badolato R, Wang JM, Stornello SL, Ponzi AN, Duse M, Musso T. Serum amyloid A is an activator of PMN antimicrobial functions: induction of degranulation, phagocytosis, and enhancement of anti-Candida activity. *J. Leukoc. Biol.* 2000;67(3):381-6.

Bolscher JG, van der Kraan MI, Nazmi K, Kalay H, Grün CH, Van't Hof W, Veerman EC, Nieuw Amerongen AV. A one-enzyme strategy to release an antimicrobial peptide from the LFampin-domain of bovine lactoferrin. *Peptides.* 2006 Jan;27(1):1-9.

Chen HL, Yen CC, Lu CY, Yu CH, Chen CM. Synthetic porcine lactoferricin with a 20-residue peptide exhibits antimicrobial activity against *Escherichia coli*, *Staphylococcus aureus*, and *Candida albicans*. *J. Agric. Food Chem.* 2006;54(9):3277-82.

Djeu JY, Liu JH, Wei S, Rui H, Pearson CA, Leonard WJ, Blanchard DK. Function associated with IL-2 receptor-beta on human neutrophils. Mechanism of activation of antifungal activity against *Candida albicans* by IL-2. *J. Immunol.* 1993;150(3):960-70.

Dong J, Yu H, Zhang Y, Diao H, Lin D. Soluble fusion expression and characterization of human beta-defensin 3 using a novel approach. *Protein Pept. Lett.* 2011;18(11):1126-32.

Edgerton M, Koshlukova SE. Salivary histatin 5 and its similarities to the other antimicrobial proteins in human saliva. *Adv. Dent. Res.* 2000;14:16-21.

Goldman IL, Georgieva SG, Gurskiy YG, Krasnov AN, Deykin AV, Popov AN, Ermolkevich TG, Budzevich AI, Chernousov AD, Sadchikova ER. Production of human lactoferrin in animal milk. *Biochem. Cell Biol.* 2012;90(3):513-9.

Guthmiller JM, Vargas KG, Srikantha R, Schomberg LL, Weistroffer PL, McCray PB Jr, Tack BF. Susceptibilities of oral bacteria and yeast to. *Antimicrob. Agents Chemother.* 2001;45(11):3216-9.

Haney EF, Nazmi K, Bolscher JG, Vogel HJ.Structural and biophysical characterization of an antimicrobial peptide chimera comprised of lactoferricin and lactoferrampin. *Biochim. Biophys. Acta.* 2012;1818(3):762-75.

Håversen L, Kondori N, Baltzer L, Hanson LA, Dolphin GT, Dunér K, Mattsby-Baltzer I.Structure-microbicidal activity relationship of synthetic fragments derived from the antibacterial alpha-helix of human lactoferrin. *Antimicrob. Agents Chemother.* 2010; 54(1):418-25.

Hein M, Valore EV, Helmig RB, Uldbjerg N, Ganz T. Antimicrobial factors in the cervical mucus plug. *Am. J. Obstet. Gynecol.* 2002;187(1):137-44.

Jiang Y, Yi X, Li M, Wang T, Qi T, She X. Antimicrobial activities of recombinant mouse β-defensin 3 and its synergy with antibiotics. *J. Mater. Sci. Mater. Med.* 2012;23(7): 1723-8.

Jones EM, Smart A, Bloomberg G, Burgess L, Millar MR. Lactoferricin, a new antimicrobial peptide *J. Appl. Bacteriol.* 1994;77(2):208-14.

Kasetty G, Papareddy P, Kalle M, Rydengård V, Mörgelin M, Albiger B, Malmsten M, Schmidtchen A. Structure-activity studies and therapeutic potential of host defense peptides of human thrombin *Antimicrob. Agents Chemother.* 2011;55(6):2880-90.

Kondori N, Baltzer L, Dolphin GT, Mattsby-Baltzer I. Fungicidal activity of human lactoferrin-derived peptides based on the antimicrobial αβ region. *Int. J. Antimicrob. Agents.* 2011;37(1):51-7.

Lin P, Wong JH, Ng TB. A defensin with highly potent antipathogenic activities from the seeds of purple pole bean. *Biosci. Rep.* 2009;30(2):101-9.

López-García B, Lee PH, Yamasaki K, Gallo RL. Anti-fungal activity of cathelicidins and their potential role in *Candida albicans* skin infection. *J Invest Dermatol.* 2005;125(1):108-15.

Lupetti A, Danesi R, van 't Wout JW, van Dissel JT, Senesi S, Nibbering PH. Antimicrobial peptides: therapeutic potential for the treatment of Candida infections. *Expert Opin. Investig. Drugs.* 2002;11(2):309-18.

McLean DT, Lundy FT, Timson DJ. IQ-motif peptides as novel anti-microbial agents. *Biochimie.* 2013;95(4):875-80.

Okuda D, Yomogida S, Kuwahara-Arai K, Hitamatsu K, Tamura H, Nagaoka I. Augmentation of the antimicrobial activities of guinea pig cathelicidin CAP11-derived peptides by amino acid substitutions *Int. J. Mol. Med.* 2009;23(4):501-8.

Okutomi T, Tanaka T, Yui S, Mikami M, Yamazaki M, Abe S, Yamaguchi H. Anti-Candida activity of calprotectin in combination with neutrophils or lactoferrin. *Microbiol. Immunol.* 1998;42(11):789-93.

Palma C, Cassone A, Serbousek D, Pearson CA, Djeu JY. Lactoferrin release and interleukin-1, interleukin-6, and tumor necrosis factor production by human polymorphonuclear cells stimulated by various lipopolysaccharides: relationship to growth inhibition of *Candida albicans*. *Infect. Immun.* 1992;60(11):4604-11.

Palma C, Serbousek D, Torosantucci A, Cassone A, Djeu JY. Identification of a mannoprotein fraction from *Candida albicans* that enhances human polymorphonuclear leukocyte (PMNL) functions and stimulates lactoferrin in PMNL inhibition of candidal growth. *J. Infect. Dis.* 1992;166(5):1103-12.

Peyrin-Biroulet L, Beisner J, Wang G, Nuding S, Oommen ST, Kelly D, Parmentier-Decrucq E, Dessein R, Merour E, Chavatte P, Grandjean T, Bressenot A, Desreumaux P, Colombel JF, Desvergne B, Stange EF, Wehkamp J, Chamaillard M. Peroxisome proliferator-activated receptor gamma activation is required for maintenance of innate antimicrobial immunity in the colon. *Proc. Natl. Acad. Sci. USA.* 2010;107(19):8772-7.

Pusateri CR, Monaco EA, Edgerton M. Sensitivity of *Candida albicans* biofilm cells grown on denture acrylic to antifungal proteins and chlorhexidine. *Arch. Oral Biol.* 2009; 54(6):588-94.

Schroeder BO, Wu Z, Nuding S, Groscurth S, Marcinowski M, Beisner J, Buchner J, Schaller M, Stange EF, Wehkamp J. Reduction of disulphide bonds unmasks potent antimicrobial activity of human β-defensin 1. *Nature.* 2011;469(7330):419-23.

Semlali A, Leung KP, Curt S, Rouabhia M. Antimicrobial decapeptide KSL-W attenuates Candida albicans virulence by modulating its effects on Toll-like receptor, human β-defensin, and cytokine expression by engineered human oral mucosa. *Peptides.* 2011;32(5):859-67.

Sharma H, Nagaraj R. Antimicrobial activity of human β-defensin 4 analogs: insights into the role of disulfide linkages in modulating activity. *Peptides.* 2012;38(2):255-65.

Shi Y, Song W, Feng ZH, Zhao YT, Li F, Tian Y, Zhao YM. Disinfection of maxillofacial silicone elastomer using a novel antimicrobial agent: recombinant human beta-defensin-3. *Eur. J. Clin. Microbiol. Infect. Dis.* 2009;28(4):415-2.

Tran D, Tran P, Roberts K, Osapay G, Schaal J, Ouellette A, Selsted ME. Microbicidal properties and cytocidal selectivity of rhesus macaque theta defensins. *Antimicrob. Agents Chemother.* 2008;52(3):944-53.

Turner J, Cho Y, Dinh NN, Waring AJ, Lehrer RI. Activities of LL-37, a cathelin-associated antimicrobial peptide of human neutrophils. *Antimicrob. Agents Chemother.* 1998; 42(9):2206-14.

Umazume M, Ueta E, Osaki T. Reduced inhibition of *Candida albicans* adhesion by saliva from patients receiving oral cancer therapy. *J. Clin. Microbiol.* 1995;33(2):432-9.

van der Does AM, Bogaards SJ, Ravensbergen B, Beekhuizen H, van Dissel JT, Nibbering PH. Antimicrobial peptide hLF1-11 directs granulocyte-macrophage colony-stimulating factor-driven monocyte differentiation toward macrophages with enhanced recognition and clearance of pathogens. *Antimicrob. Agents Chemother.* 2010;54(2):811-6.

van der Kraan MI, van der Made C, Nazmi K, van't Hof W, Groenink J, Veerman EC, Bolscher JG, Nieuw Amerongen AV. Effect of amino acid substitutions on the candidacidal activity of LFampin 265-284. *Peptides.* 2005;26(11):2093-7.

Vasudevan S, Yuan J, Osapay G, Tran P, Tai K, Liang W, Kumar V, Selsted ME, Cocco MJ. Synthesis, structure, and activities of an oral mucosal alpha-defensin from rhesus macaque. *J. Biol. Chem.* 2008;283(51):35869-77.

Venkatesh MP, Pham D, Kong L, Weisman LE. Prophylaxis with lactoferrin, a novel antimicrobial agent, in a neonatal rat model of coinfection. *Adv. Ther.* 2007;24(5):941-54.

Venkatesh MP, Rong L. Human recombinant lactoferrin acts synergistically with antimicrobials commonly used in neonatal practice against coagulase-negative staphylococci and *Candida albicans* causing neonatal sepsis. *J. Med. Microbiol.* 2008; 57(Pt 9):1113-21.

Viejo-Díaz M, Andrés MT, Fierro JF. Different anti-Candida activities of two human lactoferrin-derived peptides, Lfpep and kaliocin-1. *Antimicrob. Agents Chemother.* 2005;49(7):2583-8.

Viejo-Díaz M, Andrés MT, Fierro JF. Modulation of *in vitro* fungicidal activity of human lactoferrin against *Candida albicans* by extracellular cation concentration and target cell metabolic activity. *Antimicrob. Agents Chemother.* 2004;48(4):1242-8.

Vorland LH, Ulvatne H, Andersen J, Haukland H, Rekdal O, Svendsen JS, GuttebergTJ. Lactoferricin of bovine origin is more active than lactoferricins of human, murine and caprine origin. *Scand. J. Infect. Dis.* 1998;30(5):513-7.

Wakabayashi H, Abe S, Okutomi T, Tansho S, Kawase K, Yamaguchi H. Cooperative anti-Candida effects of lactoferrin or its peptides in combination with azole antifungal agents. *Microbiol. Immunol.* 1996;40(11):821-5.

Wakabayashi H, Okutomi T, Abe S, Hayasawa H, Tomita M, Yamaguchi H. Enhanced anti-Candida activity of neutrophils and azole antifungal agents in the presence of lactoferrin-related compounds. *Adv. Exp. Med. Biol.* 1998;443:229-37.

Yamamoto D, Shinohara Y, Nagadome H, Terada Y. Development of tissue conditioner capable of binding with anti-microbial protein lactoferrin. *J. Prosthodont. Res.* 2009;53(3):136-41.

Yamane ES, Bizerra FC, Oliveira EB, Moreira JT, Rajabi M, Nunes GL, de Souza AO, da Silva ID, Yamane T, Karpel RL, Silva PI Jr, Hayashi MA. Unraveling the antifungal activity of a South American rattlesnake toxin crotamine. *Biochimie.* 2013 Feb; 95(2):231-40.

Ye J, Zhao H, Wang H, Bian J, Zheng R. A defensin antimicrobial peptide from the venoms of *Nasonia vitripennis*. *Toxicon.* 2010;56(1):101-6.

Yen CC, Shen CJ, Hsu WH, Chang YH, Lin HT, Chen HL, Chen CM. Lactoferrin: an iron-binding antimicrobial protein against *Escherichia coli* infection. *Biometals.* 2011; 24(4):585-94.

Zanetti M, Gennaro R, Romeo D. Cathelicidins: a novel protein family with a common proregion and a variable C-terminal antimicrobial domain. *FEBS Lett.* 1995;374:1-5.

In: Candida *albicans*: Symptoms, Causes and Treatment Options ISBN: 978-1-62808-882-3
Editors: Leon A. Dietrich and Tim S. Friedmann

Chapter V

Antifungal Therapy of Candidiasis with Amphotericin B: New Formulation for an Old Drug

Lamia Belkherroubi-Sari*

Laboratoire Antibiotiques antifongiques: physicochimie synthèse et activité biologique.
University of Tlemcen, Tlemcen. Algeria

Abstract

Amphotericin B (AmB) remains the reference treatment for invasive fungal infections and the current guidelines for the treatment of haematogenous candidiasis recommend the use of AmB. Despite the diversity of antifungal drugs to cure these infections, only the action of AmB spectrum covers most of the *Candida* organisms, which are pathogenic species to humans. In addition, the cost of the treatment is an important element in the therapeutic strategy as fluconazole, voriconazole, and caspofungin are significantly more expensive than AmB. The conventional AmB-deoxycholate (Fungizone®) formulation which is a colloidal suspension of AmB has been available since 1958. While AmB is relatively cheaper, it has a large number of adverse effects, such as renal toxicity which constitutes the main reason for its restricted use. This toxicity is partially reduced with the antifungal lipid formulations. Unfortunately, their high cost (up to 90 times more expensive than Fungizone®) limits greatly their use in clinics and particularly in poor countries. To overcome this problem, some solutions have been proposed. However after exposure yeast cells to AmB, they were in a dormant state for 24 hours then the cells regrowth. Dormancy is one of the causes that reduce the effectiveness of the antifungal strategy. New formulation of amphotericin B based on the modulation of the physicochemical environment of the drug is discussed in this chapter in order to enhance the therapeutic index of amphotericin B.

* Corresponding author: lamiabio@yahoo.fr.

1. Introduction

Fungi have recently emerged as a frequent cause of opportunistic infections worldwide. *Candida* and *Aspergillus* species are the most frequently encountered causes of fungal infections, followed by *Cryptococcus neoformans* and the Zygomycetes; all are associated with high morbidity and mortality. Overall, the incidence of candidemia and invasive candidiasis is 10 to 15 fold higher than invasive aspergillosis [73].

Candida species are opportunistic fungal pathogens that have become a major cause of nosocomial infections [47]. *Candida* bloodstream infections have become a major problem in tertiary care hospitals worldwide. Candidemia is observed particularly among patients hospitalized for long periods who have been exposed to broad-spectrum antimicrobial chemotherapy, immunosuppressive therapy, parenteral nutrition, and invasive medical procedures [27]. Moreover, both solid organ transplant (SOT) and hematopoietic stem cell transplant (HSCT) recipients are at high risk for invasive fungal infections (IFI) due to risk factors including long-term central venous catheter use, immunosuppression, and cytopenia, as well as therapy given to prevent graft-versus-host disease or rejection. *Candida* species are the leading cause of invasive fungal infections in SOT patients, causing 53% of fungal infections, and the second leading cause of invasive fungal infections in HSCT patients, causing 28% of infections [58].

Most of the manifestations of candidiasis are associated with the formation of biofilms at a wide range of implanted medical devices like catheters. In addition, the resistance of *C. albicans* biofilms is a multifactorial phenomenon [34] because biofilms escape the immune response [64] and significantly reduce the sensitivity to antifungal therapy [1]. On the other side, one distinct characteristic of *C. albicans* is its ability to produce chlamydospores that are formed on the ends of elongated suspensor cells attached to hyphae, and as it is known, the chlamydospore is a distinctive morphological feature of the fungal pathogen *C. albicans* that can be formed in nutrient depletion and oxygen-limited environments. The role of chlamydospores in the normal life cycle or pathogenicity of *C. albicans* is about to be established and this structure was rarely observed in tissue samples [29].

Amphotericin B (AmB) remains the reference treatment for invasive fungal infections and the current guidelines for the treatment of haematogenous candidiasis recommend the use of AmB [36]. Despite the diversity of antifungal drugs to cure these infections, only the action of AmB spectrum covers most of the *Candida* organisms, which are pathogenic species to humans [24, 67]. In addition to this, the cost of the treatment is an important element in the therapeutic strategy as fluconazole, voriconazole, and caspofungin which are significantly more expensive than AmB [45, 51]. The conventional AmB-deoxycholate (Fungizone®) formulation, which is a colloidal suspension of AmB, has been available since 1958. While AmB is relatively cheaper, it has a large number of side effects, such as renal toxicity which constitutes the main reason for its restricted use. AmB hence poses a serious toxicity problem in clinical practice, and it is essential to find a way for increasing the therapeutic index.

AmB toxicity is partially reduced with the antifungal lipid formulations [2]. Unfortunately, their high cost (up to 90 times more expensive than Fungizone®) [60] limits greatly their use in clinics and particularly in poor countries. To overcome this problem, some solutions have been proposed, including heating Fungizone® at 70°C for 20 minutes [37, 38], or preparation of a polyaggregate AmB obtained by the solubilization of the antifungal in a solution containing sodium deoxycholate [36,59] which allows a reduction of toxicity while retaining the effectiveness. proposed. However, after exposing yeast cells to AmB, they were in a dormant state for 24 h, and then the cells re-grew [22]. Dormancy is one of the causes that reduce the effectiveness of the antifungal strategy.

But before going further, it is necessary to understand the basic mechanisms of toxicity joining the mechanisms of action of amphotericin B, which are known to be related to the physicochemical characteristics of the molecule amphotericin B.

2. Physical and Chemical Properties of Amphotericin B

Amphotericin B is an antibiotic isolated from a culture of *Streptomyces nodosus* whose structure was established in 1970. It is part of the macrolide family (cyclic molecule closed by an internal ester bond) polyene [43]. Its molecular weight is 960 [25]. It includes a rigid apolar part made of seven conjugated double bonds responsible for the lipophilicity of the molecule and an intense absorption spectrum that allows spectroscopic studies. One rigid pole portion consisting of seven hydroxyl groups. It also includes the mycosamine witch is an amino sugar (figure 1).

Requires the rigid chain structure in the molecule sticks, with one face hydrophilic and the other face is hydrophobic, limiting considerably the solubility of the molecule in an aqueous medium. It is poorly soluble in non-polar organic solvents such as alcohols and esters, but soluble in polar organic solvents such as dimethyl sulfoxide (DMSO) and dimethyl formamide (DMF) or the alcoholic solutions [43]. The insolubility of this compound in an aqueous medium is responsible for basic phenomena of toxicity, hence the necessity to find formulations more soluble [30].

3. Mechanisms of Action of Amphotericin B

The mechanism of action of amphotericin B the most widely accepted is that proposed by De Kruijif and Demel [32]. According to their model, amphotericin B has a high affinity with membrane sterols (both ergosterol fungal cells as cholesterol animal cells) where the formation of complexes AmB/sterol. In fact, there are three hydrogen bonds between the β-OH sterols (which play role as proton acceptors) and the amino group of amphotericin B (which acts as a donor proton) [55, 61]. Each complex is associated with the formation of transmembrane channels that drain ions and metabolites, which causes cell death [62, 69]. However, the affinity of amphotericin B for ergosterol is greater than for cholesterol [68]. The steric conformation of ergosterol is more favorable than that of cholesterol to establish links between this type of sterol and the amphotericin B [20, 21, 46]. Moreover, it appeared that amphotericin B induced ion permeability potassium through membranes containing cholesterol at a certain threshold concentration [15].

The equilibrium between monomers and aggregates plays a important role in the activity of the drug. The toxicity of amphotericin B toward membranes containing ergosterol is observed at concentrations where amphotericin B is entirely in monomeric form. It would be capable of join the ergosterol present in the membrane fungal cells, which lead to the formation of channels. However, it appears that the leakage induced potassium with amphotericin B in membrane cholesterol and more particularly in the red blood cell, only occurs when amphotericin B is in the form of oligomers [13].

The lytic mechanism of amphotericin B is then based on the formation of channels in the ionic membrane; these channels are formed from 4 to 12 monomer units' amphotericin B [41]. These insoluble oligomers amphotericin B is due to the electrostatic interaction between the NH^{3+} and COO^{-} molecules antifungal adjacent one hand, and the other intramolecular hydrogen bonds part [6, 52]. Other studies highlight the role of membrane phospholipids. In fact amphotericin B interaction-sterol dependent on membrane composition phospholipids [28]. Cells of *Saccharomyces cereviciae* enriched in phospholipids such phosphatidylcholine (PC), phosphatidylethanolamine (PE) and phosphatidylserine (PS), develop resistance to amphotericin B (Rao T.V.G. et al., 1985). The interaction between phospholipids and amphotericin B reduces the free concentration of the antifungal reduced its therapeutic action [42]. On the other hand, NH^{3+} of amphotericin B form hydrogen bonds with the PO^{4-} dimiristoyl ofphosphatidylcholine lipid bilayers. Each of these interactions is responsible for the creation of a complex amphotericin B/phospholipid. In this case, sterols are only changing the membrane fluidity and helps amphotericin B to take the appropriate orientation necessary for the formation of channels. [5, 31].

In addition to the ability to form pores through the plasma membrane, amphotericin B peroxide lipid [19, 70], and inhibits the action of membrane enzymes such as ATPase proton *Candida* or Na^{+}/K^{+} ATPase of erythrocytes [14]. In another hand, in serum amphotericin B is essentially in a form bound to lipoproteins [18] and very little in free form. In this case amphotericin B will not only bind to the membranes of mammalian cells but be internalized by endocytosis [74]. Studies have shown that is by setting amphotericin B to low density lipoprotein (LDL), which have membrane receptors that are specific to them, that the internalization of amphotericin B will be [54, 75].

4. Physicochemical Environment and Amphotericin B

Amphotericin B usually administered, marketed under the name of Fungizone®, is an aqueous suspension associated with the deoxycholate of sodium. However, its use remains delicate because of its nephrotoxicity dose-dependent and its acute toxicity related to the perfusion at type of nausea, vomiting or fever [53]. Since these past 10 years, the progress made in the development of new formulas galenic, have able it to reduce its toxicity while maintaining its clinical effectiveness. Firstly the derivatives of amphotericin B, they are obtained by making chemical changes on the parent molecule in order to increase its solubility in the aqueous environment. Twenty derivatives of amphotericin B have been prepared. The groupement carboxyl terminus of the macrolide serves as a basis for the preparation of esters and amides, whereas the grouping amine of the mycosamine is employed for the preparation of the N-acyl, N-guanidine, N-methyl, N-glycosyl and N-aminocyl [12, 26, 49].

One of the derivatives of amphotericin B the most promising is the N-(1-piperidinepropionyl) amphotericin B methyl ester (PAME).It is obtained by chemical substitution of the amino group and the carboxylic group of the parent molecule. This PAME strongly reduces the *in vitro* toxicity of amphotericin B. In addition, the antifungal effectiveness toward *Candida albicans* is maintained in these conditions [42].

The formulations the most promising are the lipid forms. The principle of amphotericin B lipid rests on the preferential capture by the reticulo-endothelial tissues with gradual release of amphotericin B, more particularly at the site of infection. This mode of transfer of the amphotericin B protects the cells of the body, in particular the kidney cells. These compounds are different in term of physicochemical structure, size, pharmacokinetics, behavior in biological environment and toxicity [39].The lipid formulations of amphotericin B marketed currently in the world are: amphotericin B lipid complex (Abelcet®), liposomal amphotericin B (Ambisome®) and amphotericin B colloidal dispersion(Amphocil®, Amphotec®)[4]. Unfortunately, these lipid formulations have a cost price importing what limits significantly their use in poor country.

All these various formulations (lipid and derived) lead a reduction of the toxicity of the amphotericin B to cells hosts. This reduction of the toxicity is bound on one hand to an increase of the solubility of the molecule of amphotericin B, on the other hand it is essentially bound to the state of aggregation of the antifungal in these various formulations.

So whatever is the mechanism of action or the pharmacological activity, the toxicity of the amphotericin B depend strongly on the molecular organization of the amphotericin B in the various formulations [38].

Let us call back that in aqueous solution amphotericin B is a mixture of species that is, soluble monomers, water-soluble self-associated and water-non soluble aggregates [56]. Studies have shown that the soluble and non soluble aggregates of amphotericin B are the most toxic towards animal cells, although the water-non soluble aggregate of AmB is less toxic [30, 37, 44]. Besides, the lipid forms of the amphotericin B serve to convey the least toxic forms of the amphotericin B towards the animal cells [57, 66]. Moreover the state of aggregation of the amphotericin B molecule can be modulated by the physicochemical environment, e.g. temperature, light, ionic strength and pH [5, 33, 35, 48, 72].

5. Amphotericin B, Ionic Strength and pH

Concerning the ionic strength and the amphotericin B, it is known that the divalent metal ions affect the interaction between antifungal polyenic and the cells. Indeed, previous research has shown that magnesium and calcium disturb the effect of nystatin and amphotericin B on erythrocytes [16] and on *Saccharomyces cerevisiae* [7, 17]. In the presence of AmB salts play a significant role in the activity of this drug. According to the Hofmeister theory, salts can modify the physicochemical properties of water: ions known as "kosmotropic" increase solubility in water, whereas ions known as "chaotropic" reduce solubility [3, 76]. The kosmotropic anions, such as sulfate, citrate, or phosphate, reduce the solubility of amphotericin B in aqueous medium, thus valorizing the oligomeric forms, whereas the chaotropic anions, such as thiocyanate and trichloracetate, completely solubilize AmB and its derivatives [72]. Moreover, an increase of ionic force decreases the concentration of the monomers of amphotericin B 3-dimethylaminopropylamid [11] and of *N*-methyl-*N*-fructosyl amphotericin B methyl-ester (MFAME) [71]. However the toxicity of AmB toward the animal cells is not modulated by the ionic environment of the antifungal one. Although the carbonates allowed a significant improvement in the therapeutic index of amphotericin B [23], the significant shift of pH (from 5.6±0.2 to 8.3±0.2) caused by their addition to the culture medium is a major disadvantage, as the pH is also a significant factor in the modulation of antifungal activity [8]. Moreover only $MgCl_2$ protects the human red blood cell from the toxic effect of amphotericin B; the erythrocytes lose only 30% of their K^+. This salt increases the effectiveness of the amphotericin B against *C albicans* by 10% [23].

In vitro study showed that at pHs 5.4 or 10.8 amphotericin B stock solution reduce significantly the toxicity toward the red blood cells [8] and the *in vivo* testingrevealed that the injection of a solution of amphotericin B at 1 mg/kg, solubilized at pH 5.4 does not cause significant blood parameter disturbances in renal urea-creatinin or liver transaminase-alkaline phosphatase in Wistar rats. However, at pH 10.8, it induces significant serum urea, creatinin, alkaline phosphatase and transaminase modification. For the treatment of Wistar rats infected with the yeast *Candida albicans*, the solution of amphotericin B, solubilized at pH 5.4 used at 0.5 mg/kg every 24 hours seems to be totally effective after 7 injections (negative blood)[9].

Heated conventional Fungizone® at 70°C during 20 minutes allows a reduction of cell toxicity [63], because after heating the antifungal solution, molecules of AmB formed super aggregates which are the less toxic species towards animal cells [37]. Toxicity of Fungizone® (amphotericin B deoxycholate of sodium) is also dependant of these parameters. Heating the antifungal stock solution prepared at pH 5.4 during 20 minutes at 70°C induces only 5% of hemolysis after 120 minutes of incubation, which is the same rate observed with conventional Fungizone® heated 20 min at 70°C [10]. However amphotericin B activity toward fungal cells develops in three steps. First, all cells sustain strong perturbations that result in a marked shrinking. Then, for a long period that can extend over 24 h, no change appears. Finally, a number of cells resume activity and growth, and it may be assumed to have been in a ''dormant'' state [22]. The remainder of cells without activity may be assumed to be dead cells. Dormancy is the term which describes this intervening period, and is defined as a reversible state of low activity, where cells can persist for extended periods without division [50], which corresponds exactly to what have observed with stock solutions of Fungizone® prepared under various conditions of pHs and temperature. The logarithmic growth phase began between 23 and 26 hours of incubation at 30°C. Furthermore, these stock solutions prepared at pH5.4 inhibited yeast growth between 50 and 75% (versus 100% of growth with conventional Fungizone®) after 30 hours of culture growth [10].

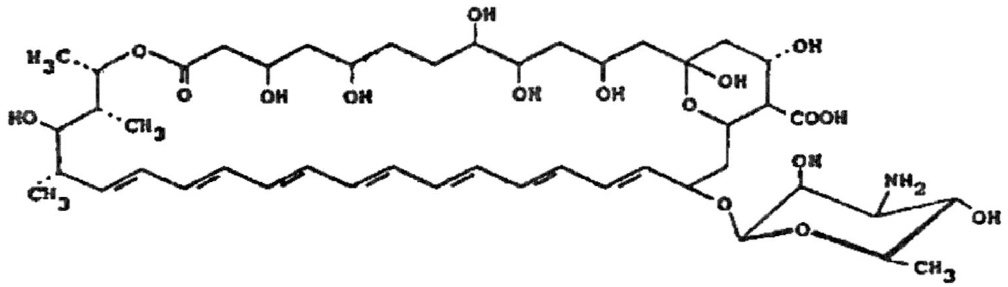

Figure 1. Structure of amphotericin B [40].

Conclusion

Yeast dormancy was one of the causes in the failure of antifungal therapy. So the growth phase of microorganisms might be considered in the planning of dosage protocols with Fungizone®, particularly with *C. albicans* infections. The preparation of a new formulation of Fungizone® from a stock solution buffered at pH 5.4 and heated during 20 minutes at 70°C seems to be a possible solution in the treatment of invasive candidiases which allows an increase of therapeutic index of Fungizone®.

References

[1] Al-Dhaheri, R. S. & Douglas, L. J. (2008). Absence of amphotericin B-tolerant persister cells in biofilms of some *Candida* species. *Antimicrob Agents Chemother*, *52*,1884-1887.

[2] Alvarez-Lerma, F., Mariscal, F., Quintana, E., Rialp, G., Diaz-Reganon, J., Perez San José, M. J. & coll. (2010). Impact of the administration of liposomal amphotericin B in patients with renal function impairment at initiation of treatment. *Journal of Chemother*, *22*, 285-287.

[3] Amore, A., Roccatello, D., Picciotto, G., Emancipator, S. N., Ropolo, R., Cacace, G., Suriani, A., Gianoglio, B., Massimino, L. S., Cirina, P., Mazzucco, G., Alfieri, V., Piccoli, G., Coppo, R. & De Filippi, P. (1997). Processing of IgA Aggregates in a Rat Model of Chronic Liver Disease. *Clinical Immunology and Immunopathology*, *84*, 107-114.

[4] Andrès, E., Tiphine, M., Letscher-Bru, V. & Herbrecht, R. (2001). Nouvelles formes lipidiques de l'amphotéricine B Revue de la littérature. *Rev Méd Interne*, *22*, 141-150.

[5] Aseandei A. & Luchian T. (2008). Ion selectivity, transport properties and dynamics of amphotericin B channels studied over a wide range of acidity changes. *Colloids and Surfaces Biointerfaces*, *67*, 99–106.

[6] Baginski, M., Resat, H. & McCammon J. A. (1997). Molecularproperties of amphotericinB membrane channel: a molecular dynamics simulation. *Mol. Pharmacol*, *52*, 560-570

[7] Beezer, A. E., Chowdry. (1980). Flow microcolorimetric bioassay of polyene antibiotics:interaction with growing *Saccharomyces cerevisiae*. *Experientia*, *37*, 828

[8] Belkherroubi-Sari, L., Boucherit, Z., Chéron, M., Boucherit, K., Benyoucef, M. & Belbraouet, S. (2008). Modulation of the polyene antibiotic amphotericin B selective toxicity by pH change of the stock solutions. *African J Microbiol Res*, *2*, 242-246.

[9] Belkherroubi-Sari, L., Boucherit, Z., Boucherit, K. & Belbraouet, S. (2011). Study of renal toxicity in Wistar rats following the action of amphotericin B solution prepared under extreme pH conditions. *Food Nutr Sci*, *2*, 731-5.

[10] Belkherroubi-Sari, L., Adida, H., Seghir, A., Boucherit, Z. & Boucherit, K. (2013). New strategy for enhancing the therapeutic index of Fungizone®. *Journal de Mycologie Médicale*, *23*, 3-7.

[11] Blanc, I., Bueno Da Costa, M. H., Bolard, J. & Saint-Pierre Chazalet, M. (2000). Oligonucleotide delivery by a cationic derivative of the polyene antibiotic amphotercin

B: Interaction oligonucleotide/vector as studied by optical spectroscopy and electron microscopy. Biochim. *Biophys. Acta*, *1464*, 299-308.

[12] Bolard, J. (1991). Mechanism of action of an anti-*Candida* drug: amphotericin B and its derivatives. Ed. R. Prasad, 214-23.

[13] Bolard, J., Legrand, P., Heitz, F. & Cybulska, B. (1991). One-sided action of amphotericin B on cholesterol-containing membranes is determined by its self-association in the medium. *Biochemistry*, *30*, 5707-5715.

[14] Bolard, J. & Vertut-Doï, A. (1995). Internalisation of amphotericin B and other polyene antifungals in mammalian cells: a possible origin of their toxicity. *Drug transport of antimicrobial and anticancer chemotherapy*. Marcel Dekhar Inc, 307-325.

[15] Bolard, J., Joly, V. & et Yeni, P. (1997). Amphotéricine B: ancien médicament, nouveaux concepts. *Médecine thérapeutique*, *3* (3), 207-213.

[16] Brajtburg, J., Medoff, G., Kobayashi, G. S., Elberg, S. & Finegold, C. (1980). Permeabilizing and hemolytic action of large and small polyene antibiotics on human erythrocytes. Antimicrob. *Agents Chemother*, *18*, 586-592.

[17] Brajtburg, J., Medoff, G., Kobayashi, G. S. & Elberg, S. (1980). Influence of extracellular K^+ or Mg^{2+} on the stages of antifungal effects of amphotericin B and filipin. Antimicrob. *Agents Chemother*, *18*, 593-597.

[18] Bratjburg, J., Elberg, S., Bolard, J., Kobayashi, G. S., Levy, R. A., Ostlund, R. E. Jr., Schlessinger, D. & Medoff, G. (1984). Interaction of plasma proteins and lipoproteins with amphotericin B. *J. Infec. Dis*, *149*, 986-997.

[19] Bratjburg, J., Elberg, S., Schwartz, D. R., Vertut-Croquin, A., Schlessinger, D., Kobayashi, G. & Medoff, G. (1985). Involvement of oxydative damage in erythrocyte lysis induced by amphotericin B. Antimicrob. *Agents and Chemother*, *27* (2), 172-176.

[20] Bratjburg, J., Powderly, W. G., Kobayashi, G. S. & Medoff, G. (1990). Amphotericin B : current understanding of mechanisms of action. Antimicrob. *Agents and Chemother*, *34* (2), 183-188.

[21] Bratjburg, J., Powderly, W. G., Kobayashi, G. S. & Medoff, G. (1990). Amphotericin B delivery systems. Antimicrob. *Agents and Chemother*, *34* (3), 381-384.

[22] Boucherit, Z., Seksek, O. & Bolard, J. (2007). Dormancy of *Candida albicans* cells in the presence of the polyene antibiotic amphotericin B: simple demonstration by flow cytometry. *Med Mycol*, *45*, 525-33.

[23] Boucherit, K., Boucherit, Z., Belkherroubi-Sari, L. & Belbraouet, S. (2010) Effect of the ionic environement of the therapeutic index of amphotericin B. *Chemical Technology*, *6* (1), 18-23.

[24] Canuto, M. M. & Rodero, F. G. (2002). Antifungal drug resistance to azoles and polyenes. *Lancet Infect Dis*, *2*, 550-63.

[25] Carbon, C., Regnier, B., Saimot, G., Valide, J. L. & Yeni, P. (1994). Antifungiques: données générales. Ed. *Médecine Science Flammarion*, 449-461.

[26] Chéron, M., Cybulska, B., Mazerski, J., Grzybosvska, J., Czerwinski, A. & Borowski, E. (1988). Quantitative structure-activity relationships in amphotericin B derivatives. *Biochem. Pharmacol.*, *37*, 827-836.

[27] Cisterna, R., Ezpeleta, G., Telleria, O., Guinea, B., Garcia Rodriguez, J. & coll. (2010). Nationwide sentinel surveillance of bloodstream *Candida* infections in tertiary care hospitals in Spain. *Journal of clinical microbiology*, *48*, 4200-4206.

[28] Clejan, S. & Bittman, R. (1985). Rates of amphotericin B and filipin association with sterols : a study of changes in sterol structure and phospholipid composition of vesicules. *The journal of biological chemistry*, *260* (5), 2384-2889.

[29] Cole, G. T., Seshan, K. R., Phaneuf, M. & Lynn, K. T. (1991). Chlamydospore-like cells of Candida albicans in the gastrointestinal tract of infected, immunocompromised mice. *Can J Microbiol*, *37*, 637-46.

[30] Cybulska, B., Bolard, J., Seksek, O., Czerwinski, A. & Borowski, E. (1995). Identification of the structural elements of amphotericin B and other polyene macrolide antibiotics of the heptane's group influencing the ionic selectivity of the permeability pathways formed in the red cell membrane. Biochim. *Biophys. Acta*, *1240*, 167-178.

[31] Czub, J. & Baginski, M. (2006). Modulation of amphotericin B membrane interaction by cholesterol and ergosterol-a molecular dynamics study, *J. Phys. Chem. B*, *110*, 16743-16753.

[32] De Kruijf, B. & Demel, R. A. (1974). Polyene antibiotic–sterol interactions in membranes of Acholeplasma laidlawii cells and lecithin liposomes. III. Molecular structure of the polyene antibiotic–cholesterol complexes. Biochim. *Biophys. Acta*, *339*, 57-70.

[33] Dupont, G., Rinnert, H. & Lematre, J. (1977). Etude physico-chimique de l'amphotéricine B en milieu alcalin. *Compte Rendu de l'académie des sciences Paris*, *284*, 853-856.

[34] Donlan, R. M. (2001). Biofilm formation: a clinically relevant microbiological process. *Clin Infect Dis*, *33*, 1387-92.

[35] Ernst, C., Dupont, G., Rinnert, H. & et Lematre, J. (1978). Effet des variations de température sur le dichroïsme circulaire, le spectre d'absorption et la diffusion Rayleigh de l'amphotéricine B en solution aqueuse et hydroalcoolique. *Compte Rendu de l'académie des sciences Paris*, *286*, 175-178.

[36] Espada, R., Valdespina, S., Dea, M. A., Molero, G., Ballesteros, M. P., Bola, F., et al. (2008). In vivo distribution and therapeutic efficacy of a novel amphotericin B poly-aggregated formulation. *J Antimicrob Chemother*, *61*, 1-7.

[37] Gaboriau, F., Cheron, M., Petit, C. & Bolard, J. (1997). Heat-induced super aggregation of amphotericin B reduces its in vitro toxicity: a new way to improve its therapeutic index. *Antimicrob Agents Chemother*, *41*, 2345-51.

[38] Gagos′, M., Herec′, M., Arczewska, M., Czernel, G., Dalla Serra, M. & Gruszecki, W. I. (2008). Anomalously high aggregation level of the polyene antibiotic amphotericin B in acidic medium: implications for the biological action. *Biophys Chem*, *136*, 44-9.

[39] Germaud, P., Morin, O. & et Moreau, P. (2001). Antifongiques et aspergilloses. *Revue Française des Laboratoires*, *332*, 31-36.

[40] Gray, K. C., Palacios, D. S., Dailey, I., Endo, M. M., Uno, B. E., Wilcock, B. C. & Burke, M. D. (2012). Amphotericin primarily kills yeast by simply binding ergosterol. *Proceeding of the National Academy of Sciencies of the united state of America (PNSA)*, *109* (7), 2234-2239.

[41] Gruszecki, W. I., Gagos, M., Herec, M. & Kernen, P. (2003). Organization of antibiotic amphotericin B in model lipid membranes. A mini review, *Cell. Mol. Biol. Lett.*, *8*, 161-170.

[42] Hąc-Wydro, K., Dynarowicz-Łątka, P., Grzybowska, J. & Borowsk, E. (2005). *N*-(1-Piperidinepropionyl)amphotericin B methyl ester (PAME)—a new derivative of the

antifungal antibiotic amphotericin B: Searching for the mechanism of its reduced toxicity, *Journal of Colloid and Interface Science*, *287*, 476-484.

[43] Hammond, S. M. (1977). Biological activity of polyene antibiotics. *Progress in medical chemistry*, (*14*). Edd. G. P. Bllis and G. R. West:106-164.

[44] Hargreaves, P. L., Nguyen, T. S. & Ryan, R. (2006). Spectroscopic studies of amphotericin B solubilized in nanoscale bilayer membranes. *Biochimica et Biophysica Acta*, *1758*, 38–44.

[45] Hennequin, C., Gauzit, R., Wolff, M. & Cordonier, C. (2010). Recommandations de stratégies thérapeutiques pour le traitement des candidoses et aspergilloses invasives chez l'adulte. *Infections Fongiques Antifongiques*, *12*, 165-170.

[46] Herve, M., Debouzy, J. C., Borowski, E., Cybulska, B. & Gary-Bobo, C. M. (1989). The role of the carboxyl and amino groups of polyene macrolides in their interactions with sterols and their selective toxicity. A ^{31}P-NMR study. Biochim. *Biophis. Acta*, *980*, 261-272.

[47] Hsu, D. I., Nguyen, M., Nguen, L., Law, A. & Wong-Beringer, A. (2010). A multicentrique study to evaluate the impact of caspofungin administration on outcomes of invasives candidiasis in non-immunocompromised adult patients. *Journal of antimicrobial chemotherapy*, *65*, 1765-1770

[48] Hung, C. T., Lam, F. C., Perrier, D. G. & Souter, A. (1988). A stability study of amphotericin B in aqueous media using factorial design. *Int J Pharm*, *44*, 117-23.

[49] Jarzebsky, A., Falkowski, L. & Borowski, E. (1982). Synthesis and structure-activity relationships of amides of amphotéricine B. *J. Antibiot.*, *35*, 220-229.

[50] Kaprelyants, A. S. & Kell, D. B. (1993). Dormancy in stationary-phase culture of *Micrococcus luteus*: flow cytometric analysis of starvation and resuscitation. *Appl Environ Microbiol*, 3187-3196.

[51] Kettani, A., Belkhadir, Z. H., Mosadik, A., Faroudy, A., Ababou, A., Lazreq, A., et al. (2006). Traitement antifongique des candidoses systémiques en réanimation. *J Mycol Med*, *16*,16-25.

[52] Khutorsky, V. (1996). Ion coordination in the amphotericin B channel, *Biophys. J., 71*, 2984-2995.

[53] Kleinberg, M. (2006). What is the current and future status of conventional amphotericin B? *International Journal of Antimicrobial Agents*, *27*, 12–16.

[54] Koldin, M. K., Kobayashi, G. S., Bratjburg, J. & Medoff, G. (1985). Effects of elevation of serum cholesterol and administration of amphotericin B complexed to lipoproteins on amphotericin B-induced toxicity in rabbits. Antimicrb. *Agents and Chemother*. *28*, 144-148.

[55] Lance, M. R., Washington, C. & Davis S. S. (1996). Evidence for the formation of amphotericin B-phospholipid complexes in Langmuir monolayers. *Pharm. Res.*, *13*, 1008-1014.

[56] Legrand, P., Romero, E. A., Cohen, E. & Bolard, J. (1992). Effects of aggregation and solvent on the toxicity of amphotericin B to human erythrocytes. *Antimicrob Agents Chemother*, *36*, 2518-2522.

[57] Legrand, P., Vertut-Doi, A. & Bolard, J. (1996). Comparative internalization and recycling of different amphotericin B formulations by a macrophage-like cell line. *J. Antimicrob Chemother*, *37*, 519-533.

[58] Lockhart, S. R., Wagner, D., Iqbal, N., Pappas, P. G., Andes, D. R.,Kauffman, C. A., Brumble, L. M., Hadley, S., Walker, R. & coll. (2011). Comparison of in vitro susceptibility characteristics of *Candida* species from cases of invasive candidiasis in solid organand stem cell transplant recipients: Transplant-Associated Infections Surveillance Network (TRANSNET), 2001 to 2006. *J Clin Microbiol, 49*, 2404–2410.

[59] Mariné, M., Espada, R., Torrado, J., Pastor, F. J., Guarro, J. (2008). Efficacy of a new formulation of amphotericin B in a murine model of disseminated infection by *Candida glabrata*. *J Antimicrob Chemother, 61*, 1-4.

[60] Martino, R. (2004). Efficacy, safety and cost-effectiveness of amphotericin B lipid complex (ABLC): a review of the literature. *Curr Med Res Opin, 20*, 485-504.

[61] Mazerski, J., Grzybowska, J. & Borowski, E. (1990). Influence of net charge on the aggregation and solubility behaviour of amphotericin B and its derivatives in aqueous media. Eur. *Biophys J., 18*, 159-164.

[62] Mazerski J., Bolard J. & Borowski E. (1995). Effect of the modifications of ionizable groups of amphotericin B on its ability to form complexes with sterols in hydroalcoholic media. Biochim. *Biophys. Acta., 1236*, 170–176.

[63] Petit, C., Cheron, M., Joly, V., Rodrigues, J. M., Bolard, J. & Gaboriau, F. (1998). *In-vivo* therapeutic efficacy in experimental murine mycoses of a new formulation of deoxycholate-amphotericin B obtained by mild heating. *J Antimicrob Chemother, 42*, 779-85.

[64] Ramage, G., Saville, S. P., Thomas, D. P. & Lopez-Ribot, J. L. (2005). *Candida* biofilms: an update. *Eukaryot Cell, 4*, 633-8.

[65] Rao, T. V. G., Trivedi, A. & Prasad, R. (1985). Phospholipid enrichment of *Saccharomyces cereviciae* and its effect on polyene sensitivity. Can. *J. Microbiol., 31*, 322-326.

[66] Ridente, Y., Aubard, J. & Bolard, J. (1999). Absence in amphoteicin B-spiked human plasma of free monomeric drug, as detected by SERS. *FEBS letter, 12* (446), 283-286.

[67] Sanglard, D. & Odds, F. C. (2002). Resistance of *Candida* species to antifungal agents: molecular mechanisms and clinical consequences. *Lancet Infect Dis, 2*, 73-85.

[68] Seoane, R., Minones, J., Conde, O., Casas, M. & Iribarnergaray E. (1998). Molecular organisation of amphotericin B at the air-water interface in the presence of sterols : a monolayer study. Bichim. *Biophys. Acta, 1375*, 73-83.

[69] Seoane, R., Minones, J., Conde, O., Casas, M. & Iribarnegaray, E. (1999). Interaction between amphotericin B and sterols in monolayers mixed films of ergosterol–amphotericin B, *langmuir, 15*, 3570-3578.

[70] Sokol-Anderson, M. L., Bratjburg, J. & Medoff, G. (1986). Amphotericin B-induced oxydative damage and killing of *Candida albicans*. *J. Infec. Dis., 154*, 76-83.

[71] Szindler-Reichert, J., Mazerski, J., Cybulska, B., Grzyboska, J. & Borowski, E. (2001). MFAME, *N*-methyl-*N*-D-fructosyl amphotericin B methyl ester, a new amphotericin B derivative of low toxicity : relationship between self-association and effects on red blood cells. Biochim. *Biophys. Acta, 1528*, 15-24.

[72] Toledo Grijalba, M., Chéron, M., Borowski, E., Bolard, J. & Schreier, S. (2006). Modulation of polyene antibiotics self-association by ions from the Hofmeister series. *Biochimica and Biophysica Acta., 1760*, 973-979.

[73] Vazquez, J. A. (2010). Invasive fungal infections in the intensive care unit. *Seminars in respiratory and critical care medicine, 31*(1), 79-86.

[74] Vertut-Doï, A., Ohnishi, S. I. & Bolard, J. (1994). The endocytic process in CHO cells, a toxic pathway of the polyene antibiotic amphotericin B. Antimicrob. *Agents and Chemother. 38*, 2373-2379.

[75] Wasan, K. M., Rosenblum, M. G., Cheun, L. & Lopez-Berestein, G. (1994) Influence of lipoproteins on renal cytotoxicity and antifungal activity of amphotericin B. Antimicrob. *Agents and Chemother*, *38*, 223-227.

[76] Washabaugh, M. W. & Alins, K. D. (1983). Purification of aqueous ethylene glycol. *Analytical Biochemistry*, *134*, 144-152.

In: Candida *albicans*: Symptoms, Causes and Treatment Options ISBN: 978-1-62808-882-3
Editors: Leon A. Dietrich and Tim S. Friedmann

Chapter VI

Candida albicans Infection in Cases of Lower Respiratory Tract Infections among HIV/AIDS Patients in Calabar, Nigeria

***O. M. Ogba*[1,*], *L. N. Abia-Bassey*[2] *and J. Epoke*[2]**
[1]Department of Medical Microbiology/Parasitology,
University of Calabar Teaching Hospital, Calabar, Nigeria
[2]Department of Medical Laboratory Science, University of Calabar, Nigeria

Abstract

Background: *Candida albicans* is the the most pathogenic of about 68 species of *Candida*. It is a member of the normal flora of the skin, mucuos membranes, and gastrointestinal tract. *Candida* pneumonia is one of the most challenging of all the *Candida* infections. Primary *Candida* pneumonia refers to infections limited to the lungs, while secondary *Candida* pneumonia indicates lung involvement due to the movement of invasive *Candida* from other parts of the body.

Symptoms: The major clinical manifestations of primary *Candida* pneumonia are fever and tachypnoea. Radiologically, nonspecific patchy infiltrates can be seen. The only accepted criterion for the definitive diagnosis of *Candida* pneumonia is histological demonstration of the fungus in the lung.

Causes: Respiratory *Candida* infection can result from exogenous or endogenous source, hematogenous spread or by introduction of the pathogen into the lungs via catheters and lines.

Treatment options: Several factors must be considered when choosing antifungal agents for patients with HIV/AIDS. One important factor is efficacy. Antifungals are less efficacious in HIV-positive patients than in patients with cancer, and time for antifungal response is also more prolonged. In addition the relapse rate is higher in patients with

*Corresponding author: Ogba, Ofonime Mark, E-mail: ofonimemark@yahoo.com, Phone: +2348035404728.

HIV than in other patient's populations. Fluconazole is one of the most effective agents for the treatment of pulmonary candidiasis, especially in patients with AIDS. Fluconazole is active against most *Candida* species; however, resistant *C. albicans* strains have been isolated, primarily from AIDS patients under prolonged fluconazole treatment.

Aims and objectives: This study was designed to identify and characterize *Candida albicans* isolated from lower respiratory tract infections of HIV positive patients and to determine the prevalence rates of *Candida* infections among these subjects.

Materials and methods: Two early morning expectorate sputum samples were collected from 272 HIV positive subjects visiting the ART clinics and DOTS centre with cases of lower respiratory tract infection, over a period of 14 months from May, 2009 - July 2010 in Calabar. Subjects were recruited for this study upon approval by the Ethical Research Committee of the University of Calabar Teaching Hospital and obtaining written informed consent from the patients. Samples were processed by standard methods for isolation of *Candida*. Speciation was done by germ tube test, chlamydospore production on corn meal agar and sugar fermentation and assimilation tests using the Microexpress Candida identification kit (Tulip, India).

Results: Out of the 544 sputum samples collected from 272 subjects, *Candida* species were isolated from 40 (14.7%) and identified after confirming their growth in the second sample. The majority of *Candida* species among the *Candida* isolates were *Candida albicans* (80%) followed by *Candida tropicalis* 5(12.5%), *Candida dublinensis* 2(5.0%) and *Candida guilliermondii* 1(2.5%). The isolation rate of *Candida albicans* from sputum samples was found to be highest among subjects aged 25-34 years, followed by those aged 15-24 years. This study is the first of its kind to be carried out in Calabar and the South-South geopolitical region of Nigeria, and has shown that pulmonary albicans candidiasis is a health problem among HIV positive patients in Calabar.

Background

Candida albicans is the most common fungal pathogen, and is the organism responsible for the majority of localized fungal infections in humans. Contributing to its high degree of association with disease is its high prevalence in the healthy population. It is a member of the normal flora of the mucous membranes in the gastrointestinal, upper respiratory and female genital tracts. It is the species most commonly isolated from nearly all forms of candidiasis [1, 2]. Patients with impaired immunity, such as those who have AIDS or are neutropenic as a result of cancer therapy, are at particular risk of developing *C. albicans* infections,which may become systemic. *Candida* species are ubiquitous fungi and are the most common fungal pathogens that affect humans. The growing problem of mucosal and systemic candidiasis reflects the enormous increase in the number of patients at risk and the increased opportunity that exists for *Candida* species to invade tissues normally resistant to invasion. *Candida* species are true opportunistic pathogens that exploit recent technological advances to gain access to the circulation and deep tissues [3].

The increased prevalence of local and systemic disease caused by *Candida* species has resulted in numerous new clinical syndromes, the expression of which depends primarily on the immune status of the host. *Candida* species produce a wide spectrum of diseases, ranging from superficial mucocutaneous disease to invasive illnesses, such as hepatosplenic candidiasis, *Candida* peritonitis, and systemic candidiasis [4].

Advances in medical technology, chemotherapeutics, cancer therapy, and organ transplantation have greatly reduced the morbidity and mortality of life-threatening disease but patients who are critically ill and in medical and surgical ICUs have been the prime targets for opportunistic nosocomial fungal infections, primarily due to *Candida* species. Studies suggest that the problem is not under control and, in fact, show it is worsening. On a daily basis, virtually all physicians are confronted with a positive *Candida* isolate obtained from one or more various anatomical sites. High-risk areas for *Candida* infection include neonatal, pediatric, and adult ICUs, both medical and surgical. *Candida* infections can involve any anatomical structure [5].

Introduction

Genus Candida

The heterogeneous genus *Candida* belongs to the family Cryptococcaceae within the Deuteromycetes (Fungi Imperfecti) [6]. *Candida* is a polymorphic fungus. It is a Gram positive, oval, budding yeast cell that produces pseudohyphae both in culture and in tissues and exudates [7]. They exhibit filamentous mycelial morphology in the saprophytic phase, but have typical yeast morphology in the parasitic phase, in tissue and when grown at 37°C in the laboratory [7]. They form pseudohyphae when the buds continue to grow but fail to detach, producing chains of elongated cells that are pinched or constricted at the septations between cells [8]. At temperatures below 26°C in nutritionally poor media such as cornmeal agar, it produces thick-walled resting cells 7 to 17mm in diameter, called chlamydospores [9]. There are about 68 species of *Candida* and the most pathogenic is *C. albicans* [1]. The other non-albicans Candida (NAC) species includes; *C. dubliniensis, C. glabrata, C. guilliermondii, C. tropicalis, C. parapsilosis, C. krusei and C. hisitaniae, C. kefyr, C. lipolytic and C. pelliculos* [10, 11].

Candida pnuemonia

Candida pneumonia is one of the most challenging of all the *Candida* infections. Primary *Candida* pneumonia refers to infections limited to the lungs, while secondary *Candida* pneumonia indicates lung involvement due to the movement of invasive *Candida* from other areas of the body [12]. The criteria for the diagnosis of pulmonary candidiasis are still controversial. The isolation of Candida from culture of sputum, endotracheal aspirates, bronchoscopic samples, percutaneous lung needle aspirates and even from lung tissue may only represent colonization of the trachea-bronchial tree (1). Despite the debate about the diagnosis of pulmonary candidiasis, the definitive diagnosis still rest on histological demonstration of the yeast in lung tissue with associated inflammatory changes at autopsy [14, 15].

The increase in the number of immunocompromised patients during the last few decades, as a result of chemotherapy or HIV/AIDS has resulted in a parallel increase in the number of opportunistic infections, especially those due to *Candida* species [16, 17].

Rapid identification and speciation of *Candida* species is essential in clinical laboratories. However, no single phenotypic test is highly effective in identifying *Candida* species and combination of tests is sometimes necessary for identification. Although molecular techniques employed to characterize *Candida* species are sensitive and specific, it is not cost effective for routine clinical mycology laboratories in resource constrained setup like ours [18].

Pathophysiology

Candida species are confined to human and animal reservoirs; however, they are frequently recovered from the hospital environment, including foods, countertops, air-conditioning vents, floors, respirators, and medical personnel. They are also normal commensals of diseased skin and mucosal membranes of the gastrointestinal, genitourinary, and respiratory tracts [19].

Candida species also contain their own set of well-recognized but not well characterized virulence factors that may contribute to their ability to cause infections [20].
The main virulence factors include the following:

- Surface molecules that permit adherence of the organism to other structures (e.g., human cells, extracellular matrix, prosthetic devices)
- Acid proteases and phospholipases that involve penetration and damage of cell envelopes
- Ability to convert to a hyphal form (phenotypic switching)

As with most fungal infections, host defects also play a significant role in the development of candidal infections. Host defense mechanisms against *Candida* infection and their associated defects that allow infection are as follows:

- Intact mucocutaneous barriers - Wounds, intravenous catheters, burns, ulcerations
- Phagocytic cells
- Polymorphonuclear leukocytes - Chronic granulomatous disease
- Monocytic cells -Myeloperoxidase deficiency
- Complement -Hypocomplementemia
- Immunoglobulins -Hypogammaglobulinemia
- Cell-mediated immunity - Chronic mucocutaneous candidiasis, diabetes mellitus, cyclosporin A, corticosteroids, HIV infection
- Mucocutaneous protective bacterial florae - Broad-spectrum antibiotics [20].

Risk factors associated with invasive or systemic candidiasis include the following: Granulocytopenia, bone marrow transplantation, solid organ transplantation (liver, kidney), parenteral hyperalimentation, hematologic malignancies, foley catheters, solid neoplasms, recent chemotherapy or radiation therapy, corticosteroids, broad-spectrum antibiotics, burns, prolonged hospitalization, severe trauma, recent bacterial infection, recent surgery, gastrointestinal tract surgery, central intravascular access devices, premature birth, hemodialysis, acute and chronic renal failure and mechanical ventilation for longer than 3 days [21].

The first step in the development of a candidal infection is colonization of the mucocutaneous surfaces. All of the factors outlined above are associated with increased colonization rates. The routes of candidal invasion include (1) disruption of a colonized surface (skin or mucosa), allowing the organisms access to the bloodstream, and (2) persorption via the gastrointestinal wall, which may occur following massive colonization with large numbers of organisms that pass directly into the bloodstream [22].

Epidemiology

Respiratory *Candida* infections involving the lungs or bronchial system appear predominantly in patients with underlying primary diseases, like HIV/AIDS [23]. Bronchopneumonia can originate from hematogenous spread of the fungus as part of a disseminated infection or from introduction of the pathogen into the lung [1]. The diagnosis of pulmonary candidiasis is difficult not because it is difficult to demonstrate the organism in clinical samples but because isolation of *Candida* species in sputum does not necessarily mean that a person is suffering from pulmonary candidiasis. A good clinical correlation is therefore necessary to ascertain the clinical significance of the isolate (4).

Candida species globally remain the most frequently implicated opportunistic fungal pathogens in HIV/AIDS infection [13] probably because they are endogenous opportunists, and were the most prevalent fungal agent in our study [26], occurring in 14.7% (40/272) of HIV-positive patients. These results are in agreement with the 12.1% prevalence reported in India [13], but considerably lower than a 48% prevalence reported in New York, USA by Diaz-Fuentes and colleagues [14]. However, in the New York study, *Candida* was isolated from lung tissue at autopsy; which is a definitive diagnostic technique for pulmonary candidiasis. It is likely that none of their isolates were lost. In the study by Ogba et al. [26], no autopsy was carried out on dead participants 3 (1.10%), so we were not able to confirm what infection was present.

Candida albicans was the species most commonly identified in our study [26], followed in descending order of prevalence by C. *tropicalis*,C. *dubliniensis* and C. *guilliermondii* (Table 1). These *Candida* isolates were characterised to species level using germ tube test, chlamydospore production on corn meal agar and sugar fermentation and assimilation tests using the Microexpress Candida identification kit (Tulip, India) (Table 2). Aluyi and colleagues [27] in Edo state, Nigeria, found the distribution of *Candida* species to be as follows: *C. albicans* 19.0%, *C. stellatoidea* 9.2% and *C. parapsilosis* 8.2%. A multicentre surveillance study conducted in Quebec, Canada, in 2000 reported a distribution pattern for *Candida* as follows: *C. albicans* 64%, *C. tropicalis* 17%, *C. parapsilosis* 8%, *C. glabatra* 6% and *C. krusei* 2% [28]. The variation in the above finding perhaps reflects variation in the geographical distribution of different *Candida* species.

The isolation rate of *Candida* species from sputum samples was found to be highest among subjects aged 25-34 years, followed by those aged 15-24 years. No *Candida* species were isolated from subjects aged 65-74 years (Table 2). Jha et al. [9], found the isolation rates of *Candida* species to be highest among subjects in the seventh decade of life followed by the fourth and fifth decade. The high prevalence of *Candida* infection associated with the second and third decade of life in our study may be related to the high sexual activity of subjects in this age group, as HIV infection primarily occurs through heterosexual transmission in Nigeria [29].

Wadhwa et al. [24], diagnosed three out of 22 cases as *Candida* pneumonia (mean CD4 count161±73.08 cells μl^{-1}). A CD4 count of <200 cells μl^{-1} and a viral load of>10,000 copies ml^{-1}, along with factors like tobacco consumption, poor oral hygiene and xerostomia, have been shown to facilitate the occurrence of oral lesions in these individuals[25]. Ogba et al. [26], isolated 32/272 (11.8%) of *Candida albicans* from HIV patients with respiratory infections, with a mean CD4 count of 134.7+74.8 cells μl^{-1} of blood, the other *Candida* infections accounted for 8/272 (2.9%) cases, with mean CD4 count ranging from 49.0±0.0 to 105.0±103.2 cells/μl of blood.

Morbidity and Mortality

Candidemia and disseminated candidiasis: Mortality rates associated with these infections have not improved markedly over the past few years and remain in the range of 30-40%. Systemic candidiasis cause more case fatalities than any other systemic mycoses. More than a decade ago, investigators reported the enormous economic impact of systemic candidiasis in hospitalized patients. Candidemia is associated with considerable prolongation in hospital stays (70 days vs 40 days in comparable patients without fungemia). Although mucocutaneous fungal infections, such as oral thrush and *Candida* esophagitis, are extremely common in patients with AIDS, candidemia and disseminated candidiasis are uncommon [27].

Table 1. Distribution of *Candida* isolates among subjects

Candida species	No of isolates(n=272)	Percentage of isolates
Candida albicans	32	80
Candida tropicalis	5	12.5
Candida dubliniensis	2	5.0
Candida guilliermondii	1	2.5
Total	40	14.7

Table 2. Characterization of *Candida* species

Species	Urease utilisation	Melibose utilization	Lactose utilization	Maltose utilization	Sucrose utilization	Galactose utilization	Cellobiose Utilization	Inositol utilization	Xylose utilization	Dulcitol utilization	Raffinose utilization
C. albicans	-	-	-	+	-	+	-	-	+	-	-
C. dubliniensis	-	-	-	+	-	+	-	-	V		-
C. tropicalis	-	-	-	+	+	V	+	-	+	-	-
C. guilliermondii	-	+	-	-	+	V	+	-	+	+	+

KEY: + = positive; - = negative; v = variable.

Signs and Symptoms of Candida Pneumonia

Candida pneumonia is one of the most challenging of all the *Candida* infections. Primary *Candida* pneumonia refers to infections limited to the lungs, while secondary *Candida* pneumonia indicates lung involvement due to the movement of invasive *Candida* from other parts of the body [1]. The major clinical manifestations of primary candida pneumonia are fever and tachypnoea. Radiologically, nonspecific patchy infiltrates can be seen. Histopathologically, there is hemorrhage and necrosis [28]. Other signs includes: Focal pulmonary consolidation, reduced expansion, dullness to percussion and bronchial breathing; signs of bronchial obstruction, thoracic lymphadenopathy, and pleural effusion. Signs of extra-pulmonary involvement, such as skin lesions, meningitis, retinal lesions on ophthalmoscopy are also evident [29].

Laboratory Diagnosis

The criteria for the diagnosis of *Candida* pneumonia remain to be defined. Because there is no pathognomonic signs for *Candida* pneumonia, diagnosis has relied for years on detecting the presence of *Candida* in sputum or bronchoalveolar lavage fluid, and other respiratory samples [30]. However, these methods are subject to error since *Candida* is a normal inhabitant of the mouth, and can be found in sputum in 20 to 55% of normal subjects [30].

The organisms grow rapidly and readily at either room temperature or 37°C appearing 2 to 4 days as creamy, moist, flat colonies with a distinctive yeast odour [31]. The formation of germ tube in human sera in 2 to 3 hours is characteristic of *C. albicans, C.dubliniensis and C. stellatoidea* [32]. *Candida albicans* is differentiated from other pathogenic species of *Candida* by its ability to produce characteristic thick-walled chlamydospore and pseudomycelia bearing clusters of blastospores in rice-tween-80 agar, cornmeal agar, or chlamydopspore agar within 24 to 48 hours of incubation at room temperature. However, *C. stellatoidea* and *C. dubliniensis*is also share similar characteristics [32].

The interpretation of positive cultures varies with the specimen. Positive cultures from normally sterile sites are significant. To rule out the possibility of oropharyngeal colonization, a common feature among the HIV patients, those cases with plenty of pseudohyphae on smear examination are considered as significant pathogens [33].

The only accepted criterion for the definitive diagnosis of *Candida* pneumonia is histological demonstration of the fungus in the lung which is usually diagnosed at autopsy [34, 14].

Causes

Respiratory *Candida* infection can result from haematogenous spread of disseminated disease or by introduction of the pathogen into the lungs via various catheters and lines [1, 35]. Once *Candida* enters the bloodstream, either from exogenous or endogenous source, the microorganisms have to adhere to the endothelial surface of the blood vessels, before dissemination into tissues [36]. This process involves endocytosis, endothelial invasion, and response to the invading pathogen expressed in production of pro-inflammatory cytokines, such as tumor necrosis factor-alpha (TNF-a) or interleukin (IL)-6 [37]. Germ tubes are noted to be better endocytosed than blastospores [38].

Treatment Options

Several factors must be considered when choosing antifungal agents for patients with HIV or AIDS. One important factor is efficacy. Antifungals are less efficacious in HIV-positive patients than in patients with cancer, and time for antifungal response is also more prolonged [39]. In addition the relapse rate is higher in patients with HIV than in other patient's populations [40]. Active antifungal agents are used in the treatment of systemic candidiasis. Since treatment is usually of relative short duration, a risk of side effects and toxicity are not major causes of concern in absorbed and non-absorbed antifungal agents [41].

Fluconazole is one of the most effective agents for the treatment of pulmonary candidiasis, especially in patients with AIDS. Fluconazole is active against most *Candida* species; however, resistant *C. albicans* strains have been isolated, primarily from AIDS patients under prolonged fluconazole treatment [42].

The management of serious and life-threatening invasive candidiasis remains severely hampered by delays in diagnosis and the lack of reliable diagnostic methods that allow detection of both fungemia and tissue invasion by *Candida* species [43]. However, there are no large clinical trial data to guide therapy for this disease [45, 46]. The invasion of the lung parenchyma by *Candida* species with resulting Candida pneumonia is a rare event with controversy surrounding this entity.

Table 3. Age and gender distribution of *Candida* species among subjects

Age (years)	Gender	*Candida* species	Total (%)
15-24	Female (F)	5 *Candida albicans*	
		2 *Candida tropicalis*	9(22.5)
	Male (M)	2 *Candida albicans*	
25-34	Female (F)	12 *Candida albicans*	
		3 *Candida tropicalis*	19(47.5)
	Male (M)	3 *Candida albicans*	
		1 *Candida guilliermondii*	
35-44	Female (F)	2 *Candida albicans*	
	Male (M)	1 *Candida albicans*	4(10.0)
		1 *Candida dubliniensis*	
45-54	Female (F)	4 *Candida albicans*	
	Male (M)	2 *Candida albicans*	7(17.5)
		1 *Candida dubliniensis*	
55-64	Female (F)	-	1(2.5)
	Male (M)	1 *Candida albicans*	
65-74	Female (F)	-	-
	Male (M)	-	
	Total		40(100)

Denotes no *Candida* species was isolated.

Observational reports and case series have shown that proven *Candida* pneumonia is associated with high mortality among patients with malignancies. No convincing data for any particular form of therapy exist. Data for laryngitis are based on small series and individual case reports. Most cases have been managed with amphotericin B therapy, but milder cases successfully managed with fluconazole therapy [43, 47].

The treatment options are: Intravenous amphotericin B or oral or intravenous fluconazole [43]. Fluconazole (an orally active triazole agent) is well established as a first-line management option for both localized and systemic *C. albicans* infections [48]. In patients with candidemia who are clinically stable and who have not recently received azole therapy, a (400 mg/d or 6 mg/kg/d) of fluconazole or caspofungin (70 mg loading dose Day 1, then 50 mg/d) or micafungin (100 mg/d) or anidulafungin (200 mg on Day 1, then 100 mg/d) is recommended [47]. In patients with candidemia who are clinically unstable and for whom identification of the Candida species in the blood is unknown, amphotericin B deoxycholate (0.6–1.0 mg/kg/d), or a lipid formulation of amphotericin B (3–5 mg/kg/d), or caspofungin (70 mg loading dose Day 1, then 50 mg/d), or micafungin (100 mg/d), or anidulafungin (200 mg on Day 1, then 100 mg/d) for initial therapy [47].

The use of an agent other than fluconazole, such as either a polyene or an echinocandin-based regimen, would also apply to hospitals where primary resistance of *C. albicans* to fluconazole is high, owing to such factors as frequent use of fluconazole for prophylaxis. This recommendation is largely based on the increasing resistance to fluconazole of non-albicans *Candida* spp, specifically, *C. glabrata* and *C. krusei*, and some *C. albicans* isolates. This recommendation specifically deals with the initial empiric treatment regimen. If the *Candida* isolate is determined to be susceptible to fluconazole, then a switch to fluconazole should be made [46].

Recommendations

Most patients with primary *Candida* pneumonia and laryngeal candidiasis should be treated with amphotericin B (0.7–1.0 mg/kg per day). In cases of secondary pneumonia associated with hematogenously disseminated infection, therapy should be directed at disseminated candidiasis, rather than at *Candida* pneumonia in particular. For candidal laryngitis, fluconazole is a suitable alternative in milder cases [44].

Conclusion and Future Prospect

Pulmonary candidiasis is a health problem among HIV positive patients in Calabar, Nigeria. Microexpress candida identification kit has been found to be useful in the identification of *Candida* to species level, as PCR is expensive and not easily accessible. Periodic study of pulmonary *Candida* infections among HIV infected patients is a present day need, to know the changing pattern in incidence of *Candida* species. For future prospects modern rapid techniques like the T2Candida test and other molecular methods which are rapid test for *Candida* infections should be employed. This may reduce patients mortality significantly by diagnosing candida pneumonia and candidemia 25 times faster than sputum and blood culture can do.

Acknowledgments

We acknowledge Prof. M. F. Useh, who made time to read through this work meticulously, with tactical and intelligent suggestions. We appreciate Mr. Usetu Uno, Mr. Obeten and Mrs Arit Onen of Lawrence Henshaw hospital for their immense assistance during sample collection.

References

[1] Segal, E. & Elad, D. (2005). Candidiasis. In: Scheld, W. M., Hooper, D. C. and Hughes, J. M. (Eds.), *Topley and Wilson's Microbiology and Microbial Infections*, *10th edition* (479-623). Washington, DC: Hodder Arnold ASM Press.

[2] Dupont, P. F. (1995). *Candida albicans*, the opportunist. A cellular and molecular perspective. *Journal of the American Pediatric Medical Association*, *85*, 104–15.

[3] McCullough, M. J., Ross, B. C. & Reade, P. C. (1996). *Candida albicans*: a review of its history, taxonomy, epidemiology, virulence attributes, and methods of strain differentiation. *International Journal of Oral and Maxillofacial Surgery*, *25*, 136–44.

[4] Vazquez, J. A. (1999). Options for the management of mucosal candidiasis in patients with AIDS and HIV infection. *Pharmacotherapy*, *19*, 76–87.

[5] Pappas, P. G., Rex, J. H. & Lee, J. (2003). A prospective observational study of candidemia: epidemiology, therapy, and influences on mortality in hospitalized adult and pediatric patients. *Clin Infect Dis.*, *37*(5), 634-43.

[6] Warren, N. G. & Hazen, K. C. (2005). In: Murray, Baron, Pfaller, Tenover &Yolken. *Manual of Clinical Microbiology*, 7th edition ASM.

[7] Chakrabati, A. & Shivaprakash, M. R. (2005). Microbiology of systemic fungal infections. *Journal of Postgraduate Medicine*, *51*, 16 – 20.

[8] Calderone, R. A. & Fronzi, W. A. (2001). Virulence of *Candida albicans*. *Trends in Microbiology*, *9*, 327.

[9] Jha, B. K., Dey, S., Tamang, M. D., Joshy, M. E., Shivananda, P. G. & Brahmadatan, K. N. (2006). Characterization of *Candida* species isolated from cases of lower respiratory tract infection. *Kathmandu University Medical Journal*, *4*(3), 290-294.

[10] Odds, F. C. (1988). *Candida and candidosis*, 2nd ed. BaillierreTindall, London, United Kingdom.

[11] Hazen, K. C., Brawner, D. L., Reisselman, M. H., Cutler, J. E. & Jutila, M. A. (1991). Differential adherence of hydrophobic and hydrophilic *Candida albicans*yeast cells to mouse tissues. *Infect. Immun*, *59*, 907-912.

[12] Soll, D. R. (2002a). *Candida* and virulence: the evolution of phenotypic plasticity.*ActaTropica*, *81*, 101.

[13] Eza, D., Cerrillo, G. & Moore, D. A. (2006). Postmortem findings and opportunistic infections in HIV positive patients from a public hospital in Peru. *Patholology Research and Practice*, *202*(11), 767-75.

[14] Diaz-Fuentes, G., Shin, C., Sy, E. R., Niazi, M. & Menon, L. (2007). Pulmonary fungal involvement in HIV-positive patients in an inner city hospital in New York. *The Internet Journal of Pulmonary Medicine*, 7(2), 1531-2984.

[15] Anaparthy, U., Bharathi, M. &Sandhya, C. (2011). Isolation and Characterisation of *Candida* Species from Oropharyngeal Secretions of HIV Positive Individuals. *NaszaDermatol Online*, *2*(3), 119-124.

[16] Binesh, L. Y. &Kalyani, M. (2011). Phenotypic Characterization of *Candida* species and their antifungal susceptibility from a tertiary care centre. *Journal of Pharmaceutical and Biomedical Sciences*, *11* (12), www.jpbms.info.

[17] Juliana, C. R. (2004). Phenotypic and Genotypic Identification of *Candida* spp. isolated from hospitalized patients. *Rev IberoamMicol*, *21*, 24 - 26.

[18] Koneman, E. W., Allen, S. D., Janda, W. M., Schreckenberger, P. C. & Winn, W.C. (1997). The role of Microbiology laboratory in the diagnosis of infectious disease: Guidelines to practice and management, In: Pfeiffer, R. P. and Magnus, B. C. (eds.), *Color atlas and text book of diagnostic microbiology, 5th edition* (69). New York: Lippincot Press.

[19] Morgan, J. (2005). Global trends in candidemia: review of reports from 1995-2005. *Curr Infect Dis Rep*, *7*(6), 429-39.

[20] Yang, Y. L. (2003). Virulence factors of *Candida* species. *J Microbiol Immunol Infect*, *36*(4), 223-8.

[21] Pappas, P. G. (2006). Invasive candidiasis. *Infect Dis Clin North Am*, *20*(3), 485-506.

[22] Pfaller, M. A. & Diekema, D. J. (2007). Epidemiology of invasive candidiasis: a persistent public health problem. *Clin Microbiol Rev*, *20*(1), 133-63.

[23] Gueteau, N; Darras, A & William, T. W. (1991). Bilateral Torulopsisglabrata Pneumonia. *Revue de Pneumologie Clinique*, *47*, 137-9.

[24] Wadhwa, A; Kaur, R; Agarwal, S. K., Shyama, J. & Bhalla, P. (2007). AIDS-related opportunistic mycoses seen in a tertiary care hospital in North India. *Journal of Medical Microbiology*, *56*, 1101-1106.

[25] Bravo, I. M., Correnti, M., Escalona, L., Perrone, M., Brito, A., Tovar, V. & Rivera, H. (2006). Prevalence of oral lesions in HIV patients related to CD4 cell count and viral load in a Venezuelan population. *Medicina Oral, Patologia Oral CirugiaBucal*, *11*, *E33-39*.

[26] Ogba, O. M., Abia-Bassey, L. N. & Epoke, J. (2013).The relationship between opportunistic pulmonary fungal infections and CD4 count levels among HIV-seropositive patients in Calabar, Nigeria. *Transactions R Soc Trop Med Hyg*, *107*, 170-175. *doi:* 10.1093/trstmh/trs025.

[27] Aluyi, H. S. A., Otajevwo, F. D. & Iweriebor, O. (2010). Incidence of pulmonary mycoses in patients with acquired immunodeficiency diseases. *Nigerian Journal of Clinical Practice*, *13*(1), 78-83.

[28] Petrosillo, N., Nicastri, E. & Viale, P. (2005). Nosocomial pulmonary infections in HIV-positive patients. *Current Oppinion on Pulmonary Medicine*, *11*(3), 231-5.

[29] Mitsunaga, T. M., Powel, A. M., Heard, N. J. & Larsen, U. M. (2005). Extramarital sex among Nigerian men, polygamy and other risk factors. *Journal of Acquired Immune Deficiency Syndrome*, *39*(4), 478-88.

[30] Mandanas, R. (2005). Fungal Pneumonia: Good overview from US perspective.*EMedicine*, *1062*,95-103.

[31] El-Ebiary, M., Torres, A., Fabregas, N., Piug, J., Gonzalez, J., Ramirez, J., del Bano, D., Hernandez, C. & Jimenez, M. T. (1997). Significance of the isolation of *Candida* species from respiratory samples in critically ill, non-neutropenic patients. *American Journal of Respiratory and Critical Care Medicine*, *156*(2), 583-590.

[32] Calderone, R. A. (2002). *Candida* and Candidiasis. *N. American Society for Microbiology*, *3*(1752), 451.

[33] Soll, D. R. (2002b). Phenotypic switching. In: Calderone, R.A. (Ed.), *Candida and candidiasis* (123-43). Washington, DC: ASM Press.

[34] Shailaja, L. A., Pai, L. A., Mathur, D. R. & Lakshmi, V. (2004). Prevalence of bacterial and fungal agents causing lower respiratory tract infections in patients with HIV infection. *Indian Journal of Medical Microbiology*, *22*(1), 28-33.

[35] Haron, E., Vartivarian, S., Anaissie, E., Dekmezian, R. & Bodey, G. (1993). Primary *Candida* pneumonia. *Medicine*, *72*(3), 137-142.

[36] Khatib, R. & Clark, J. A. (1995). Relevance of culturing *Candida* species from intravascular catheters. *Journal of Clinical Microbiology*, *33*, 1635-7.

[37] Klotz, S. A. (1992). Fungal adherence to the vascular compartment; a critical step in the pathogenesis of disseminated candidiasis. *Clinical Infectious Disease*, *14*,340-7.

[38] Orozco, A. S., Zhou, X. & Filler, S. G. (2000). Mechanism of the pro-inflammatory response of endothelial cells to *Candida albicans* infection. *Infection and Immunity*, *68*, 1134-41.

[39] Phan, O. T., Belanger, P. H. & Filler, S. G. (2000). Role of hyphal formation in interactions of *Candida albicans* with endothelial cells. *Infection and Immunity*, *68*, 3485-90.

[40] Darouiche, R. O. (1998). Oropharyngeal and esophageal candidiasis in immunocompromised patients: Treatment issues. *Clinical Infectious Diseases*, *26*, 59-274.

[41] Vazquez, J. A. (2000). Therapeutic options for the management of oropharyngeal and eosophageal candidiasis in HIV/AIDS patients. *HIV Clinical Trials*, *1*, 47-59.

[42] Kirkpatrick, C. H. (1994). Chronic Mucocutaneous candidiasis. *Journal of American Dermatology*, *31*(S2), 514 – 517.

[43] Richardson, M. D. & Warnock, D. W. (1997). *Fungal infection: diagnosis and management.* Oxford: Blackwell Science.

[44] Pappas, P. G., Rex, J. H., Sobel, J. D., Filler, S. G., Dismukes, W. E., Walsh, T. J. & Edwards, J. E. (2004). Lower Respiratory Tract Candidiasis (Pulmonary and Laryngeal Candidiasis). *Clin Infect Dis*, *38* (2), 161-189. doi: 10.1086/380796

[45] Kontoyiannis, D. P., Reddy, B. T., Torres, H. A., Luna, M., Lewis, R. E., Tarrand, J., Bodey, G. P. & Raad, II. (2002). Pulmonary candidiasis in patients with cancer: an autopsy study. *Clin Infect Dis*, *34*, 400–403.

[46] Haron, E., Vartivarian, S., Anaissie, E., Dekmezian, R. & Bodey, G. P. (1993). Primary Candida pneumonia: experience at a large cancer center and review of the literature. *Medicine*, *72*, 137–142.

[47] Limper, A. H., Knox, K. S., Sarosi, G. A., Ampel, N. M., Bennett, J. E., Catanzaro, A., Davies, S. F., Dismukes, W. E., Hage, C. A., Marr, K. A., Mody, C. H., Perfect, J. R. & Stevens, D. A. (2011). Treatment of Fungal Infections in Adult Pulmonary and Critical Care Patients. *Am J Respir Crit Care Med*, *183*, 96–128. DOI: 10.1164/rccm.2008-740.

[48] Neuenschwander, M. C., Cooney, A., Spiegel, J. R., Lyons, K. M. & Sataloff, R. T. (2001). Laryngeal candidiasi. *Ear Nose Throat J*, *80*, 138-9.

[49] Edwards, J. E., Bodey, G. P., Bowden, R. A., Buchner, T., de Pauw, B. E. & Filler, S. G. (1997). International Conference for the Development of a Consensus on the Management and Prevention of Severe Candidal Infections. *Clinical Infectious Diseases*, *25*, 43–59.

In: Candida *albicans*: Symptoms, Causes and Treatment Options ISBN: 978-1-62808-882-3
Editors: Leon A. Dietrich and Tim S. Friedmann

Chapter VII

Laboratory Diagnosis of Vulvovaginal Candidosis

***S. I. Nwadioha*[1,*], *E. O. P. Nwokedi*[1], *M. S. Odimayo*[1], *G. T. A. Jombo*[1] *and I. Onwuezobe*[2]**

[1]Department of Medical Microbiology and Parasitology, College of Health Sciences, Benue State University, Makurdi, Nigeria
[2]Department of Microbiology and Parasitology, College of Health Sciences, Uyo, Akwa ibom state, Nigeria

Abstract

Vulvovaginal candidiasis is a leading cause of abnormal vaginal discharge. Inflammation of the vagina, as in any inflammatory sexually transmitted infection, increases the risk of acquisition of HIV. The study was set to establish the importance of the laboratory support in diagnosis of vaginal candidiasis in order to improve treatment of vaginal candidiasis in current syndromic management of abnormal vaginal discharge. A finding based on a prospective study of female genital swabs in some Primary Health Care Centers in Nigeria vis-à-vis a similar study in a University Teaching Hospital in Nigeria, December 2006 to December 2009 by the same author was made. Candida species were the most predominantly isolated organisms (60%) in the female genital discharges across the patients in both the primary health care centers and university teaching hospital in Nigeria. Also, young adults of age range 21 – 30 years and pregnant mothers constitute an important risk. Laboratory support was found to be necessary for a differential diagnosis or to confirm the clinical diagnosis of vaginal candidiasis. The finding shows that the high prevalence of vuvo-vaginal candidiasis cuts across social groups and necessitates a high index of diagnostic tools which is the laboratory.

Keywords: Vaginal candidiasis, laboratory, microscopy, culture

* Phone: +234- 08056838967, E-mail: samnwa2000@yahoo.com.

Introduction

Vaginal Candidiasis is a common type of vaginitis, a gynecologic disorder that manifests with an odorless curdy white discharge ("cottage cheese") in the female lower reproductive tracts with pruritus, irritation, dysuria or dyspareunia [1]. It is a common complaint among women of different age groups in any society whether or not they are sexually active. Some studies have shown high preponderance of vaginal candidiasis in infective vaginal discharge with 42 to 52.5% isolation rate of *candida* species [1, 2].

Risk factors for vaginal candidiasis are factors that do not seem to be a direct cause of the disease, but seem to be associated in some way. Having the risk factor makes the chances of the condition higher but does not always lead to vaginal candidiasis. Also, the absence of any risk factors or having a protective factor does not necessarily guard one against vaginal candidiasis [3]. Some of the risk factors include pregnancy, poorly controlled diabetes, oral contraceptive, antibiotics, immune suppression in chronic debilitating illness like HIV, tuberculosis and cancer, douches, perfumed feminine hygiene sprays, topical antimicrobial agents, tight clothing, tight under- wears, thyroid disorders and corticosteroid [3].

Vaginal candidiasis is caused by the fungus *Candida albicans* in approximately 69 to 85% of cases, while other species such as *C. glabrata, C. krusei, C. tropicalis* and *C. stellatoidea* rarely cause vaginitis [4, 5]. *Candida* species are usually of endogenous origin and may be transmitted by sexual partners and may cause balanitis, balanoposthitis and rarely urethritis in males. *Candida spp.* are usually endogenous and can be isolated from the genital tract in up to 25% of asymptomatic healthy women of child bearing age [6]. In order for *Candida spp.* to colonize the vagina, they must first adhere to the vaginal epithelial cells and then grow, proliferate and germinate, before finally causing symptomatic inflammation. Changes in the vaginal environment are usually necessary before the organism can induce pathological effects. Probably the most important defence against both colonization and inflammation is the natural bacterial flora.

The diagnosis of vaginal candidiasis can not always be established on the basis of clinical manifestations alone. Classic symptoms and signs of candidiasis include vaginal itching, an odorless curdy white discharge, a burning feeling in the vulva, dysuria, and erythema of the labia and vulva. Symptoms and signs, however, are often more equivocal. Laboratory support is necessary for a differential diagnosis or to confirm the clinical diagnosis of candidiasis. A wet-mount preparation should routinely be done not only to determine the presence of yeast cells, but also to exclude the presence of *Trichomonas vaginalis* and "clue cells". Positive direct microscopy has a very high diagnostic value. In minority of patients with symptomatic vaginal candidiasis, the microscopic examination is negative.

Culture remains the most sensitive method available for the detection of Candida. However, a positive culture does not necessarily indicate that Candida is responsible for the symptoms, as more than 20% of healthy women may harbor *Candida spp.* in the vagina [6]. Therefore, culture is only recommended if vaginal candidiasis is clinically suspected but wet-mount microscopy is negative.

Although vaginal candidiasis is both treatable and mild, when left untreated, is a possible risk for acquisition of HIV/AIDS as well as other complications [7]. Other complications include pelvic inflammatory disease, infertility, ectopic pregnancy, pelvic abscess, menstrual disorders, spontaneous abortion and premature birth [8]. It is now well established that the presence of infective vaginal discharge greatly facilitates transmission and acquisition of HIV between sexual partners [9].

Therefore, there is a need for early diagnosis and prompt treatment of this common condition especially among the risk groups, in order to avert the complications and reduce the transmission of HIV. Laboratory support is necessary for a differential diagnosis or to confirm the clinical diagnosis of vaginal candidiasis.

Collection of Specimens

Remove a sample of discharge from the vaginal wall with a swab. In general, collect the specimen from the wall of the posterior fornix. In patients who have only a slight vaginal discharge and extensive involvement of the vulva or labia, it is better to collect the specimen from the irritated mucosa. Direct microscopy can be done immediately at the clinic site or the specimen may be transported to the laboratory. The use of a transport medium, such as Amies, is not necessary if yeasts have to be identified, but is to be preferred in order to maintain viability and motility of trichomonads. This can also be ensured by placing the swab in a small tube containing 0.3 ml of saline for transport times of no more than 2 hours.

In males with balanitis, use a swab pre-moistened in saline to rub the glans of the penis.

Direct Microscopy

Place the specimen on a glass slide and, if necessary, depending on its fluidity mix a drop of saline. Cover the preparation with a coverslip and examine microscopically at X 400 magnification not only to detect yeast cells, but also to exclude the presence of trichomonads and clue cells. Yeasts are round to ovoid cells, 4 μm in diameter, showing typical budding (blastoconidia). The addition of 10% potassium hydroxide to the preparation increases slightly the detection sensitivity of yeasts, making the recognition of mycelia (pseudohyphae) much easier. In general, there is a quantitative relationship between the severity of clinical signs and symptoms and the extent of genital colonization. Yeast can easily be recognized on a Gram- stained smear as they are Gram- positive cells. The sensitivity of a wet mount, however, is superior to that of a stained smear [6].

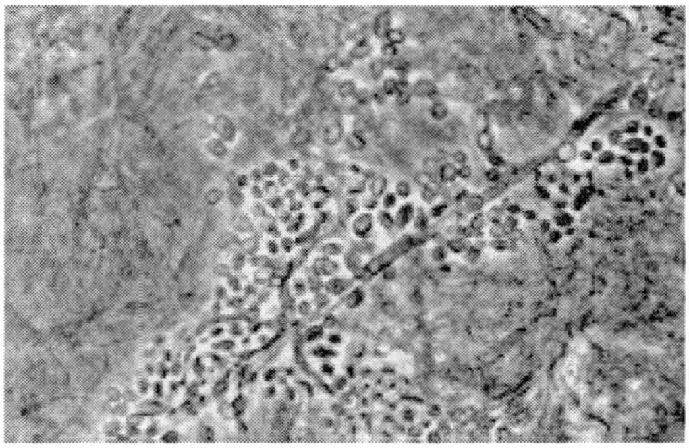

10% KOH mount showing the presence of budding yeast cells and pseudohyphae.

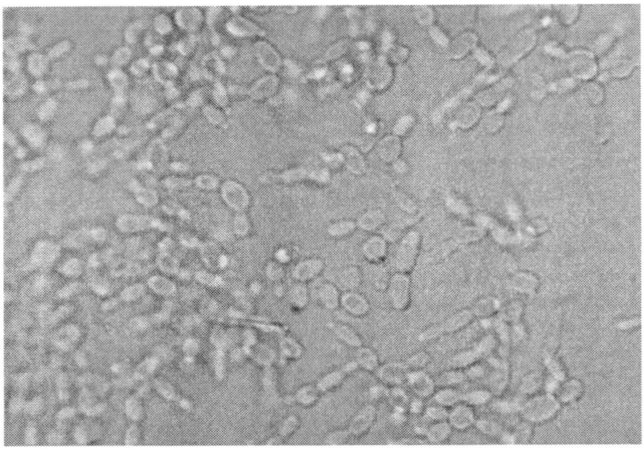

Wet Mount of Candida Budding Cells.

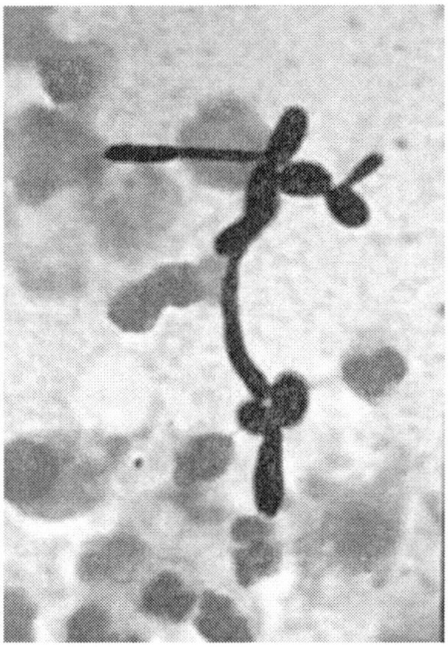

Gram Stain of Vaginal Smear.

Culture

Antibiotic treated selective Sabouraud dextrose is an excellent growth medium for isolation of *Candida spp*. After inoculation of the clinical specimen, incubate the plates at 36° C for 2 days. Yeast cells are opaque white creamy moist colonies. The only important identification for routine purposes consists of a differentiation from bacteria: pick up a colony with a bacterialological loop, suspend it in a drop of saline on a glass slide, cover with a coverslip, and examine microscopically.

Further identification of yeasts is not necessary for routine diagnosis. However, simple test for the presumptive identification of *C.albicans* is the *germ tube test.* Emulsify a colony in 0.5 ml of bovine or horse serum and incubate at 36° C for 4 hours. *C.albicans* will show short lateral hyphal filaments without any constrictions. It is examined every half an hour for formation of germ tubes. Some rare *C.albicans* do not grow germ tubes. In the past, it has been emphasized that *C. stellatoidea* also produces germ tube, and distinction between *C. albicans* should be made. Now, *C.stellatoidea* is no longer a valid species and has been combined with *C. albicans*. A complete identification of yeasts to species level can be obtained by means of auxanographic methods for carbohydrate and nitrate assimilation, or through carbohydrate fermentation tests. Kits for the identification of yeasts to species level are commercially available [6]

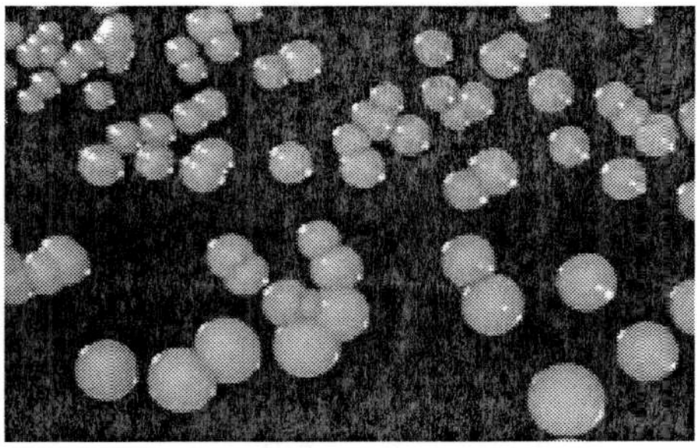

Typical moist colonies of Candida.

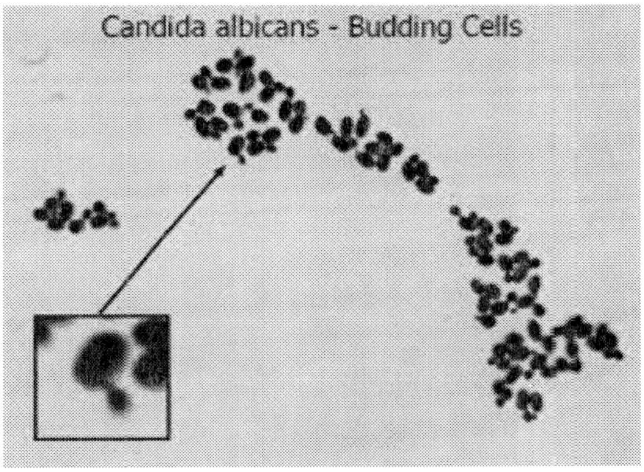

Culture Gram Stain of Budding Candida.

SPECIES	GLUCOSE	SUCROSE	LACTOSE	TREHALOSE	RAFFINOSE
C.albicans	+	+	-	+	-
C.guilliermondi	+	+	-	+	+
C. intermedia	+	+	+	+	+
C. krusei	+	-	-	-	-
C.parapsilosis	+	+	-	+	-
C. pseudotropicalis	+	+	+	-	+
C. stelloidea	+	-	-	+	-
C.tropicalis	+	+	-	+	-
C.zeylanoides	+	-	-	+	-

Sugar Assimilation Test.

Sugar Assimilation Test (Auxanogram) by Wickerham-Burton Method

Assimilation tests have largely replaced fermentation test as a means of species identification in view of equivocal fermentation test results. The method consists essentially of growing a yeast on a basal carbohydrate –free medium supplemented with the test sugar. There are many variations on the number of sugars and the method of their application to the basal medium. The following approach conveniently overcomes some of the practical problems.

a. Dispense basal medium in 10 ml amounts and autoclave.
b. While the medium is cooling, dispense about 0.5 -1mg of the test sugar into a compartment of a 10 cm square 'Repli dish'(Sterilin) which has 25 divisions. Five sugars that suffice for identification in most instances are glucose (positive control), sucrose, trahalose, lactose and raffinose. Five isolates may be tested on each plate.
c. Allow the agar medium to cool to approximately 45° C; add a few grains of powdered yeast extract to supply essential vitamins.
d. Seed the medium with 1ml of the test yeast organism from the prepared inoculum suspension.
e. Use a Pasteur pipette to distribute sufficient of the seeded medium to cover the base of each compartment. A constant depth of medium should be maintained.
f. Incubate at 30° C for 48 hours. Growth produces an opacity in the medium and indicates the ability of the isolate to assimilate a sugar. All yeasts assimilate glucose.

References

[1] Nwadioha S. I., Egah D. Z., Nwokedi E. O. P., Odimayo M. S. A study of female genital swabs in primary health care centres in Jos , Nigeria. *J. Med.* and *Pharm. sci.* 2009;5(1):95-98.

[2] Nwokedi E. E., Anyiam N. N. A study of high vaginal swabs in Kano Teaching Hospital. A preliminary report. *J. Highland Med. Res.* 2003; 1:57-61.

[3] John E. E. Mycosis. In: Mandell, Bennett and Dollin .Editors. Textbook of Principles and Practice of Infectious Diseases. 5th Ed. New York: Churchill Livingstone 2000. Pp.2291.

[4] Betty A., Forbes, Daniel F. S., Alice S. W. Editors. Genital Infections. In: laboratory manual of Bailey and Scotts diagnostic microbiology. 12th Ed. Mosby Elsevier publication 2007. Pp. 753-872.

[5] Nwadioha S. I., Nwokedi E. O. P., Egesie J., Enejuo H. Vaginal candidiasis and its risk factors among women attending a Nigerian Teaching Hospital. *The Nigerian Postgraduate Medical Journal*, 2013; 20(1):20-23.

[6] Van Dyck E., Meheus A. S., Piot P. (1999). A manual on Laboratory diagnosis of Sexually Transmitted Diseases. World Health Organization, Geneva.

[7] Nwadioha S. I., Egah D. Z., Banwat E. B., Alao O. O. Microbial agents of abnormal vaginal discharge in pregnant mothers attending PHC clinics of Jos Nigeria. *J. Clin. Med. and. Res.* 2009;2:007-011. At http//www.academicjournals.org/JCMR.

[8] Jombo G. T. A., Opajobi S. O., Egah D. Z., Banwat E. B., Denen Akaa P. Symptomatic vulvovaginal candidiasis and genital colonization by candida species in Nigeria. *J. Pub. Hlth. and Epidem.* 2010; 2(6):147-151. At http//www.academicjournals.org/JPHE

[9] Federal Ministry of Health, Department of Public Health, National AIDS/STI Control Programme. Technical report 2010: National HIV/Syphilis sero-prevalence sentinel survey among pregnant women attending antenatal clinics in Nigeria. Abuja; 2010: 1-11.

In: Candida *albicans*: Symptoms, Causes and Treatment Options ISBN: 978-1-62808-882-3
Editors: Leon A. Dietrich and Tim S. Friedmann

Chapter VIII

Symptomatology and Therapy in Candidiasis

***Reginaldo G. Lima-Neto*[1]*, Danielle P. C. Macedo*[2] *and Rejane P. Neves*[2]**
[1]Department of Tropical Medicine, Health Sciences Center, Federal University of Pernambuco (UFPE), Cidade Universitária Recife, Brazil
[2]Department of Mycology, Biological Sciences Center, UFPE, Brazil

Abstract

The yeasts are represented by several genera, including *Candida* that presents various species causing infection in humans. However, some species colonize oral cavity, vaginal mucosa and gastrointestinal tract in healthy individuals. Particularly, *C. albicans* is considered the most frequent cause of superficial infections and life-threatening systemic infections. The clinical manifestations of oral candidiasis commonly are whitish plaques strongly or weakly adhered to the mucosa. The risk factors mainly include the wearing of dentures, extremes of age, prolonged antibiotic use, and underlying diseases specially *diabetes mellitus*. This infection may to evolve into oropharynx and the esophageal candidiasis. The vulvovaginal candidiasis clinically exhibits erythematous and pruriginous lesions, white discharge and unpleasant odor. The main predisposing factors for vulvovaginal candidiasis are use of antibiotics, oral contraception, pregnancy, hormone therapy and diseases as *diabetes mellitus*. However, neutropenia and damage of the gastrointestinal mucosa are considered conditions strictly related with the development of systemic (disseminated) candidiasis. Further risk factors include invasive medical device use, which allow direct access of the yeast to the bloodstream, broad-spectrum antibiotics, surgery trauma and even disrupts mucosal barriers. Diagnosis of invasive candidiasis and candidemia remains difficult and therefore prophylactic and pre-emptive therapies appear promising strategies in high-risk patients. Currently, treatment options to superficial and deep infections include antifungal agents from four licensed different classes: I) polyenes, represented for amphotericin B and several lipid formulations besides nystatin; II) azoles that include the imidazoles cetoconazole and miconazole, in addition to triazoles fluconazole, itraconazole and newer less toxic voriconazole, posaconazole and ravuconazole; III) echinocandins anidulafungin, caspofungin and micafungin and IV) the nucleoside analogue flucytosine that is only used as a part of a combination regimen. Due to the limited armory of the available antifungal and increasing reports of resistance, the choice of combination therapy has been explored to improve healing rates and allow reduction of the dose. Important considerations when choosing the antimycotic agents include the localization of the infection, the severity of disease, depletion of organ functions, previous exposure to antifungals, the identified fungal specie and your virulence factors, local resistance patterns and patient characteristics. We review the currently available data on pathogenesis, symptomatology and management strategies for superficial and invasive candidiasis and Candidemia.

Candidiasis Symptoms

Candidiasis can cause a wide spectrum of symptoms, which can vary depending on the type of infection and clinical conditions of the patients and *Candida albicans*, the major agent of candidiasis, is commensal yeast that colonizes mucosal, oral cavities and vaginal as well as digestive tract. This microorganism may also cause a variety of infections named candidiasis which had emerged since the early 1960s. Clinically candidiasis can be distinguished in cutaneous, mucocutaneous, and also in gastrointestinal tract candidiasis, respiratory, genitourinary, hepatosplenic candidiasis and the systemic forms.

Cutaneous Candidiasis

This is a common form of candidiasis that manifests as an erytematous lesions over the intertrigo with generalized pruritus at maceration body sites. On those sites the humidity and the accumulation of organic substances provide warm and moist environments which promote the growth of *C. albicans* strains, turning a colonization conditions into a pathogenic phase. The genitocrural folds, axillae, hands and feet interdigital, retro auricular, inframammary and anal region are considered the most frequently infected body sites. At physical examination the lesions reveal a widespread rash that begins as individual vesicles spreading into large confluent areas, causing maceration and fissuring. The affected area presents a scalloped border with a white rim that surrounds the erythematous lesions.

Mucocutaneous Candidiasis

Candida infections with simultaneous damages in mucosa and skin surfaces are termed mucocutaneous candidiasis, which includes angular cheilitis, vulvovaginitis, balanopostitis, and the nail lesions.

In the angular cheilitis presentation there is an inflammatory reaction followed by painful lesions, erythema, and fissuring at the corners of the mouth, eventually with bleeding.

C. albicans is initially commensal in vagina mucosa may turn into a pathogenic yeast affecting the vulva and also the vagina, characterizing a vulvovaginitis. The symptoms are itching, burning sensation, dyspareunia and the elimination of a vaginal discharge in lumps, usually white, thick, odorless, chalky appearance. The increase of the vaginal acidity is directly related to the intensification of these symptoms. Lesions may progress to perineal, perianal and inguinal region.

In male sex this yeast may cause balanitis which affects glans penis, and frequently the prepuce. An inflammatory localized reaction is followed by symptoms including generalized erythema, irritation, swollen, soreness and may present a dry glazed appearance and a thick clumpy discharge may come from under the foreskin.

On the other hand the nail damages named onychomycosis affect especially the surrounding area (paronychia) as painful and erythematous lesions around and underneath the nail and nail bed. It is frequently diagnosed in individuals with *diabetes mellitus* and in professionals with constant immersion of the hands in water and chemical products. These clinical manifestations are associated with secondary nail thickening, ridging, discoloration, and occasional nail loss. The proximal white subungual onychomycosis is the subtype most commonly found in AIDS individuals.

In patients with an underlying genetic or immune defect leading to susceptibility to these infections, the disease is often persistent and chronic, termed chronic mucocutaneous candidiasis. This clinical presentation is severe related with persistent immunossupression conditions as endocrinopathies such as hypothyroidism, hypoparathyroidism, Addison disease, *diabetes mellitus*, thymomas, polyglandular autoimmune diseases and other underlying conditions. Simultaneous lesions affect the face, scalp, hands, nails, hair in addition to mucous membranes damages with persistent course.

Gastrointestinal Tract Candidiasis

Along the gastrointestinal tract the symptoms vary according to the different damaged sites. Thus, the oropharyngeal candidiasis frequently presents a diffuse erythema and white patches that appears on the surfaces of the buccal mucosa, throat and tongue. Commonly, the symptoms are sore and painful mouth, burning mouth or tongue, whitish thick patches on the mucosa and dysphagia.

Due to anatomic relationship of continuity, this yeast may also affect the esophageal tissue whose symptoms are: dysphagia, odynophagy, retrosternal and epigastric pain, nausea and vomiting. Less commonly, patients with underlying conditions as chronic gastric ulcerations, gastric perforations, or malignant gastric ulcers develop *C. albicans* infection.

Respiratory Tract Candidiasis

The high degree of *Candida* colonization in the respiratory tract results in candidiasis with damages in larynx, trachea, bronchi and lungs. According to the site of infection, the reported symptoms are sore throat and hoarseness, fever, productive cough, shortness of breath, respiratory distress, and different suggestive breath sounds (clear to rhonchi or scattered rales). The most common form of infection is multiple lung abscesses due to the hematogenous dissemination of *Candida* species.

Table 1. Common anti-*Candida albicans* antifungal agents

Antifungal	Dosages	Distribuition	Adverse reactions	Drug interactions	Clinical notes
Amphotericin B	IV: 0.5-0.7mg/Kg/day for total dose of 1-2g/day for 4-6 wk	Renal metabolism. Broad bioavailability. High concentrations in lungs, liver and spleen. Low concentration in *CNS.	Fever, chills, hypotension, thrombophlebitis, renal toxicity, hypokalemia and anemia.	Aminoglycosides, Antineoplastic, cyclosporine, foscarnet and pentamidine	Perform monitoring of renal markers (urea and creatinine) due to nephrotoxicity.
Ketoconazole	Oral: 200-400mg/day Topical: every 12h for 2-4 wk	Hepatic metabolism. Broad bioavailability	Hepatotoxicity, gastrointestinal impairtment, topical irritation.	Alprazolam, cisapride, midazolam, salmeterol, sirolimus, tamsulosin, terfenadine and triazolam.	No wash sites with topical application and no use antiacids, H_2-blockers and anticholinergics after 2h of oral administration.
Fluconazole	*Superficial* Oral: 50-150mg/day *Invasive* Oral: 400-800mg/day *Prophylaxis* 100-200mg in single dose one day prior surgical procedures.	Urinary clearance. Broad bioavailability. High concentrations in CNS and aqueous humor.	Nausea, vomiting, transient increase in transaminases.	Carbamazepine, cisapride, phenytoin, rifabutin, rifampicin, triazolam and warfarin	Tablet should be ingested with at least 200mL of water. No stored suspension in the freeze and to discard unused suspension after 14 days.

Antifungal	Dosages	Distribuition	Adverse reactions	Drug interactions	Clinical notes
Itraconazole	Oral: 100-400mg/day IV: 200mg every 12h	Hepatic metabolism. Broad bioavailability. Low concentrations in saliva and Urine.	Nausea, vomiting, increase in transaminases.	Astemizole, carbamazepine, cisapride, cyclosporine, digoxin, efavirenz, ergot derivatives, inhibitors of gastric acidity, levacetylmethadol, lovastatin, phenytoin, phenobarbital, pimozide, primazolam, rifampicin, simvastatin, terfenadine, triazolam and warfarin.	May to inhibit the action of oral contraceptives until 2 months posttreatment. Capsule should be ingested with food and acid drink and oral solution with empty stomach to improve absorption. Rinse mouth for a few seconds before ingesting the solution.
Voriconazole	Oral: 200mg every 12h IV: 3-6mg/kg every 12h	Hepatic metabolism. Broad bioavailability. High concentrations in CNS and Liver.	Transient visual disturbances, transient increase in transaminases, photosensitivity.	Astemizole, carbamazepine, cisapride, cyclosporine, dronedarone, efavirenz, ergot alkaloids, omeprazole, phenobarbital, quinidine, rifabutin, rifampicin, ritonavir, sirolimus, tacrolimus and terfenadine.	Administration should be carried out 1h before or 1h after meal. Prevent to operate machinery and driving at night because of visual disturbances.
Caspofungin	IV: 35-70mg/day	Broad bioavailability. Low concentrations in CNS and urine.	Fever, chills, rash, headache,anemia, hypokalemia, thrombophlebitis, hypotension, increase in transaminases, gastrointestinal impairment.	Carbamazepine, cyclosporine, dexamethasone, efavirenz, nevirapine, phenytoin and rifampin.	Dosage reduction is required in moderate hepatic impairtment.

Table 1. (Continued)

Antifungal	Dosages	Distribuition	Adverse reactions	Drug interactions	Clinical notes
Anidulafungin	*Esophageal* IV: 100mg for first day, then 50mg/day *Invasive* IV: 200mg for first day, then 100mg/day	Broad bioavailability. Low concentrations in CNS and urine.	No adverse reactions.	No drug interactions.	No adjustments necessary.
Micafungin	*Esophageal* IV: 150mg/day *Invasive* IV: 100mg/day *Prophylaxis* IV: 50mg/day	Broad bioavailability. Low concentrations in CNS and urine.	Fever, headache, hypokalemia, hypomagnesemia, neutropenia, gastrointestinal impairtment.	Itraconazole, nifedipine and sirolimus.	No adjustments necessary.

* CNS: Central nervous system.

Genitourinary Tract Candidiasis

In the genitourinary tract the *C. albicans* promotes bladder invasion resulting in frequency, urgency, dysuria, hematuria, and suprapubic pain. The evolution of cystitis may affect the upper urinary pathways and cause kidney lesions in severe cases with fever, flank pain, abdominal cramps, nausea, vomiting, chills and hematuria. In case of accumulation of fungal material in the renal pelvis occurs the urinary tract obstruction with subsequent anuria and renal insufficiency.

Systemic Candidiasis

Clinically, this presentation is classified in candidemia (*Candida* hematogenous infection) and disseminated candidiasis (deep organ infections).

During candidemia episodes occur fever unresponsive to broad-spectrum antimicrobials, nodular skin lesions (in almost 10% of patients), secondary *Candida* endophthalmitis is developed in approximately 10 to 30% of cases, with occasional sepsis and septic shock (hypotension, tachycardia, tachypnea).

The hematogenous *C. albicans* may disseminate to other organs. During bloodstream invasion or direct inoculation in surgeries this yeast commonly causes endocarditis. However, in disseminated candidiasis blood cultures are negative in up to 40-60% of patients.

As a consequence of systemic candidiasis the most frequently diagnosed symptoms and clinical presentations are renal candidiasis (commonly diagnosed at autopsy), central nervous system candidiasis (meningitis, granulomatous vasculitis, diffuse cerebritis with microabscesses, mycotic aneurysms and fever unresponsive to broad-spectrum antimicrobials), *Candida* arthritis, osteomyelitis, costochondritis, and myositis may clinically reveal tenderness over the involved area, erythema, and bone deformity, occasionally in association with a draining fistulous tract. Some patients present neutropenic and muscular pain. Other systemic clinical presentations may be diagnosed as consequence of *C. albicans* infections.

Candidiasis Causes

The infections caused by *C. albicans* commonly depend on the ability of this microorganism to grow in a range of morphological forms as yeasts, hyphae, pseudohyphae and during adverse conditions, exhibit a resistance structure (chlamydospores), enzyme production (phospolipases, proteases and keratinases), adesins and biofilms production.

The adherence of *Candida* to epithelial cells is one of the main pathogenic characteristics of the genus. Studies have shown that there are variations in the adherence capabilities of different *Candida* species, which may explain why some species colonize mucosal surfaces more frequently than others.

It is generally agreed that *C. albicans* adherence is caused by protein and carbohydrate factors and is a complicated phenomenon to study. The ALS gene family of *Candida* species encodes large cell-surface glycoproteins that are implicated in the process of adhesion to host surface. The SAP genes are another example of a gene family, which encodes secreted aspartyl proteinases, associated with pathogenicity mechanisms in *Candida* species. In addition, there is Hwpl, a developmentally regulated adhesin of germ tubes cell wall and hyphae that attaches to epithelial cells by an unconventional, transglutaminase-mediated mechanism of adhesion.

Candida albicans have been used primarily as "glycan expressing particles" to identify host cell membrane receptors. These studies have highlighted two major categories of receptors, the family of C-lectins, which specifically bind a-mannose, and a group of molecules reacting with b-glucans, initially designated as b-glucan receptors. Macrophage-mannose receptor (MR) appears to be the most representative of the receptors for mannose. MR interaction with yeasts is inhibited by α-Man. S-lectin, known as galectin-3, a 32-kDa molecule, is another receptor specific for *C. albicans* mannose and is involved in the binding of these yeasts through their cell wall β-1,2 oligomannosides. Several experiments have suggested that gal-3 is essential to the process of phagocytosis.

In addition, host favorable conditions are necessary to establishment of candidiasis. Thus, physiological factors as underlying diseases (*diabetes mellitus*, AIDS, cancer), the prolonged use of antibiotic and corticoidotherapy, surgical procedures, nutritional deficit, precarious hygiene and other factors contribute for development of this fungal infection.

Considering candidiasis as an opportunistic infection, the evaluation of risk factors in association with the nature of the underlying host defect is essential. Among the main causes of the opportunistic candidiasis are included the venous catheter, vesical catheter, prosthetic valve, parenteral nutrition and other invasive procedures.

The development of the different clinical manifestations of candidiasis may be related to pathogenic potential of the strains. Although few *Candida* species have been associated with human infections more than 200 exist in nature. The most commonly related in clinical cases is *C. albicans*, however the so called *Candida* non-*albicans* of medical importance are *C. glabrata, C. parapsilosis, C. tropicalis, C. krusei, C. kefyr, C. guilliermondi, C. lusitaniae, C. dubliniensis and C. haemulone.*

Treatment

Candida albicans is decidedly the most frequently yeast isolated of superficial and deep infections at distinct anatomical sites and in research worldwide. This species is naturally susceptible to all systemic antimycotic agents, but cases of acquired resistance to azoles have been reported in patients who have prolonged exposure to this drug class, primarily fluconazole. Furthermore, few isolates resistant to echinocandins have been also reported. Resistance to amphotericin B was previously considered anecdotal about 10-years earlier.

Treatments accomplished to manage *Candida* infections may change substantially and are guided on the anatomic location of the infection, the existence of underlying disease and immune status impaired, the presence of risk factors for infection and the susceptibility of the *Candida* isolated to specific antifungal drugs. In the last few years, there were significant changes in the management of candidiasis, particularly related to the appropriate use of echinocandins and triazoles of expanded-spectrum for candidemia and invasive candidiasis, besides mucosal candidiasis. Infectious Disease Society of America published in 2009 the newer updated guidelines to *Candida* infections.

The more recent recommendations include the echinocandins caspofungin, anidulafungin and micafungin, in addition to voriconazole and posaconazole, as well as lipid formulations of amphotericin B in several cases. Fluconazole is still considered a first-line drug to nonneutropenic patients with suspected candidemia or invasive candidiasis, although a analysis of clinical trial data comparing anidulafungin with fluconazole showed that anidulafungin was more effective in treating critically ill. Clinical trails data revised about treatment of invasive candidiasis appear to favor administration of echinocandins by increased rate of survival. This type of finding may have an impact on future treatment and strategies of drug use for candidasis in different groups of patients.

Aternative antifungal treatments may be considered who present intolerance to the treatment regimen or when the infection unresponsive to convencional antifungal therapy. The synergism of amphotericin B and flucytosine, comproved in animal models, has been used in various special situations as in immunocompromised patients with endophthalmitis, meningitis or osteomyelitis. Others combinations of antimycotics to treat complicated *Candida* infections needs to be evaluated.

Antifungal prophylaxis for candidiasis in high-risk patients is currently indicated, when stem cell transplant recipients, primarily those with allogeneic transplants, are advocated to receive fluconazole or micafungin 1 day prior of the neutropenia and continued until neutropenia resolves. Moreover, solid organ transplant may be preceded by antifungal prophylaxis with fluconazole or liposomal amphotericin B. This is recommended for postoperative antifungal prophylaxis in liver, pancreas, and small bowel transplant recipients at high risk of candidiasis. In chemotherapy-induced neutropenia, fluconazole or caspofungin is recommended for the duration of neutropenia. In addition, update of candidiasis treatment guidelines highlights the need of prophylaxis in high-risk intensive care unit patients that have presented high incidence of invasive candidiasis. Oral nystatin prevention has been recommended to decrease colonization in the patients and needs to be evaluated as a add strategy to control *Candida* related disease. Indeed, nosocomial *Candida* infection prevention must be guided on hand hygiene, optimal catheter care, and prudent antifungal administration.

In respect of research, triazoles have been extensively studied as compounds possessing important anti-*Candida* activities. A series of analogs of 1,2,3-triazoles with distinct substituents of the triazole ring have been synthesized and assessed for their antifungal activity. Modification of substituents has a great impact on the minimal inhibitory concentration values in the laboratories, since we could obtain triazole derivatives with promising activity. The antifungal tests data show that the halogen-substituted triazole derivative, mainly chlorine-substituted rings, exhibited in particular, good fungal growth inhibition, showing that further modifications can be done in order to obtain more potent prototypes.

Searches therapeutic future also should consider the knowledge of the saccharide profile of a fungal surface. Different carbohydrate specificity enables specific lectins to be selected for, therapeutic treatments, as has been proposed for cancer. Since fucose-containing structures are present on the *Candida* cell surface, it is possible that fucose-binding lectins, such *Ulex Europeus Agglutinin*, could be the basis of a therapeutic treatment of candidosis, or as a vehicle for targeted drug delivery. Furthermore, a human recombinant monoclonal antibody against heat shock protein 90 has been evaluated and displayed to improve significantly outcomes in patients treated with lipid-associated amphotericin B invasive candidiasis confirmed. However, larger randomized trials need to be performed before this combination can be used clinically.

References

Andes, D. R., Safdar, N., Baddley, J. W., Playford, G., Reboli, A. C., Rex, J. H., Sobel, J. D., Pappas, P. G., Kullberg, B. J. Impact of treatment strategy on outcomes in patients with candidemia and other forms of invasive candidiasis: a patient-level quantitative review of randomized trials. *Clinical Infectious Diseases,* 2012, v. 54, 1110-1122.

Ben-Ami, R., Garcia-Effron, G., Lewis, R. E., Gamarra, S., Leventakos, K., Perlin, D. S., Kontoyiannis, D. P. Fitness and virulence costs of *Candida albicans* FKS1 hot spot mutations associated with echinocandin resistance. *Journal of Infectious Diseases,* 2011, v. 204, 626-635.

Clancy, C. J., Nguyen, M. H. The end of an era in defining the optimal treatment of invasive candidiasis. *Clinical Infectious Diseases, 2012*, v. 54, 1123-1125.

Falcone, M., Barzaghi, N., Carosi, G., Grossi, P., Minoli, L., Ravasio, V., Rizzi, M., Suter, F., Utili, R., Viscoli, C., Venditti, M. *Candida* infective endocarditis: report of 15 cases from a prospective multicenter study. *Medicine (Baltimore)***,** 2009, v. 88, 160-168.

Fradin, C., Poulain, D., Jouault, T. Beta-1,2-linked oligomannosides from *Candida albicans* bind to a 32-kd macrophage membrane protein homologous to the mammalian lectin galectin-3. *Infection and Immunity,* 2000, v. 68, 4391-4398.

Giglio, M., Caggiano, G., Dalfino, L., Brienza, N., Alicino, I., Sgobio, A., Favale, A., Coretti, C., Montagna, M. T., Bruno, F., Puntillo, F. Oral nystatin prophylaxis in surgical/trauma ICU patients: a randomised clinical trial. *Critical Care Medicine,* 2012, v. 16, R57.

Hoyer, L. L. The ALS gene family of *Candida albicans*. *Trends Microbiology,* 2001, v. 9, 176-180.

Husain, S., Paterson, D. L., Studer, S., Pilewski, J., Crespo, M., Zaldonis, D., Shutt, K., Pakstis, D. L., Zeevi, A., Johnson, B., Kwak, E. J., McCurry, K. R. Voriconazole prophylaxis in lung transplant recipients. *American Journal of Transplantation***,** 2006, v. 6, 3008-3016.

Kett, D. H., Shorr, A. F., Reboli, A. C., Reisman, A. L., Biswas, P., Schlamm, H. T. Anidulafungin compared with fluconazole in severely ill patients with candidemia and other forms of invasive candidiasis: Support for the 2009 IDSA treatment guidelines for candidiasis. *Critical Care,* 2011, v. 15, R253.

Lima-Neto, R. G., Beltrão, E. I. C., Oliveira, P. C., Neves, R. P. Adherence of *Candida albicans* and *Candida parapsilosis* to epithelial cells correlates with fungal cell surface carbohydrates. *Mycoses,* v. 54, 23-29.

Lima-Neto, R. G., Cavalcante, N. N. M., Srivastava, R. M., Mendonça-Júnior, F. J. B., Wanderley, A. G., Neves, R. P., Anjos, J. V. Synthesis of 1,2,3-triazole derivatives and *in vitro* antifungal evaluation on *Candida* strains. *Molecules,* 2012, v. 17, 5882-5892.

Linehan S. A., Martinez-Pomares L., Gordon S. *Macrophage lectins in host defense. Microbes and Infection,* 2000, v. 2, 279-288.

Macêdo, D. P. C., Farias, A. M. A., Lima-Neto, R., Silva, V. K. A., Leal, A. F. G., Neves, R. P. Infecções oportunistas por leveduras e perfil enzimático dos agentes etiológicos. *Revista da Sociedade Brasileira de Medicina Tropical,* 2009, v.42, 188-191.

Macêdo, D. P. C., Oliveira, N. T., Farias, A. M. A., Silva, V. K. A., Wilheim, A. B., Couto, F. M., Neves, R. P. Esophagitis caused by *Candida* guilliermondii in diabetes mellitus: first reported case. *Medical Mycology,* 2010, v. 48, 862-865.

Malani, A. N., Kauffman, C. A. *Candida* urinary tract infections: treatment options. *Expert Review of Anti-infective Therapy,* 2007, v. 5, 277-284.

Maródi, L., Johnston, R. B. J. Invasive *Candida* species disease in infants and children: occurrence, risk factors, management, and innate host defense mechanisms. *Current Opinion in Pediatrics,* 2007, v. 19, 693-697.

Monod, M., Borg-Von, Z. M. Secreted aspartic proteases as virulence factors of *Candida* species. *Biological Chemistry* 2002, v. 383, 1087-1093.

Neely, L. A., Audeh, M., Phung, N. A., Min, M., Suchocki, A., Plourde, D., Blanco, M., Demas, V., Skewis, L. R., Anagnostou, T., Coleman, J. J., Wellman, P., Mylonakis, E., Lowery, T. J. T2 magnetic resonance enables nanoparticle-mediated rapid detection of candidemia in whole blood. *Science Translational Medicine,* 2013, v. 5, 182ra54.

Nurbhai, M., Grimshaw, J., Watson, M., Bond, C., Mollison, J., Ludbrook, A. Oral versus intra-vaginal imidazole and triazole anti-fungal treatment of uncomplicated vulvovaginal candidiasis (thrush). *Cochrane Database of Systematic Reviews,* 2007, CD002845.

Pach, J., Svoboda, P., Jacobs, F., Vandewoude K., van der Hoven B., Spronk P., Masterson G., Malbrain M., Aoun M., Garbino J., Takala J., Drgona L., Burnie J., Matthews R. A randomized, blinded, multicenter trial of lipid-associated amphotericin B alone versus in combination with an antibody-based inhibitor of heat shock protein 90 in patients with invasive candidiasis. *Clinical Infectious Diseases,* 2006, v. 42, 1404-1413.

Pappas, P. G. Invasive candidiasis. *Infectious Diseases Clinics of North America,* 2006, v. 20, 485-506.

Pappas, P. G., Kauffman, C. A., Andes, D., Benjamin, D. K. Jr., Calandra, T. F., Edwards, J. E. Jr. et al. Clinical practice guidelines for the management of candidiasis: 2009 update by the Infectious Diseases Society of America. *Clinical Infectious Diseases,* 2009, v. 48, 503-535.

Pfaller, M. A., Diekema, D. J. Epidemiology of invasive candidiasis: a persistent public health problem. *Clinical Microbiology Reviews,* 2007, v. 20, 133-163.

Pfaller, M. A., Pappas, P. G., Wingard, J. R. Invasive fungal pathogens: current epidemiological trends. *Clinical Infectious Diseases,* 2006, S3-S14.

Poulain, D., Jouault, T. *Candida albicans* cell wall glycans, host receptors and responses: elements for a decisive crosstalk. *Current Opinion in Microbiology,* 2004, v. 7, 342-349.

Repentigny, L., Aumont, F., Bernard, K., Belhumeur, P. Characterization of binding of *Candida albicans* to small intestinal mucin and its role in adherence to mucosal epithelial cells. *Infection and Immunity,* 2000, v. 68, 3172-3179.

Sanglard, D., Odds, F. C. Resistance of *Candida* species to antifungal agents: molecular mechanisms and clinical consequences. *Lancet Infectious Diseases,* 2002, 73–85.

Sano, H., Hsu, D. K., Apgar, J. R. et al. Critical role of galectin-3 in phagocytosis by macrophages. *Journal of Clinical Investigation,* 2003, v. 112, 389-397.

Shah, C. P., McKey, J., Spirn, M. J., Maguire, J. Ocular candidiasis: a review. *Brazilian Journal of Ophthalmology,* 2008, v. 92, 466-468.

Sharon, N., Lis, H. History of lectins: from hemagglutinins to biological recognition molecules. *Glycobiology,* 2004, v. 14, 53R-62R.

Sobel J. D. Vulvovaginal candidosis. *Lancet,* 2007, v. 369, 1961-1971.

Sundstrom, P., Cutler, J. E., Staab, J. F. Reevaluation of the role of HWP1 in systemic candidiasis by use of *Candida albicans* strains with selectable marker URA3 targeted to the ENO1 locus. *Infection and Immunity,* 2002, v. 70, 3281-3283.

Ullmann, A. J., Cornely, O. A. Antifungal prophylaxis for invasive mycoses in high risk patients. *Current Opinion on Infectious Diseases, 2006*, 571-576.

van Burik, J. A., Ratanatharathorn, V., Stepan, D. E. et al. Micafungin versus fluconazole for prophylaxis against invasive fungal infections during neutropenia in patients undergoing hematopoietic stem cell transplantation. *Clinical Infectious Diseases,* 2004, 1407-1416.

Yang, Y. L. Virulence factors of *Candida* species. *Journal of Microbiology, Immunology and Infection,* 2003, v. 36, 223-228.

In: Candida *albicans*: Symptoms, Causes and Treatment Options ISBN: 978-1-62808-882-3
Editors: Leon A. Dietrich and Tim S. Friedmann

Chapter IX

Microbial Inactivation of the Pathogen *Candida albicans* in Marine Ecosystems

***Monia El Bour*[*,1], *Imen Boukef Ben Omrane*[1] and *Abdellatif Boudabous*[2]**
[1]National Institute of Sea Sciences and Technologies – Tunisia
[2]Faculty of Mathematical, Physical and Natural Sciences of Tunis, Tunisia

Abstract

The saccharomycetes *Candida albicans* are widely distributed in marine ecosystems and their occurrence and distribution have been used as possible indicators of water pollution in the shoreline of aquatic ecosystems. Else, resistant forms of *Candida albicans* still well documented as a cause of skin infections both in human and animals and thought to be transmitted from contact with infested sands or sediments. Thus, there's actual vital interest in discovering new antimicrobial compounds with fewer environmental and toxicological risks and no resistance developped by the pathogens as *Candida albicans* and several marine natural products have been reported from large range of aquatic species with bioactivities in several species of pathogen fungi and bacteria. In present study we summarize actual data on diverse bio-activities against *Candida albicans* revealed in several species of marine algae, sponges, opistobranch mollusks and micro-epibionts.

Introduction

Fungi are chemo-heterotrophic organisms, well spread in aquatic environments and important as decomposers animal and plant, mutualistic symbionts and pathogens or spoilage organisms of natural and manufactured marine materials [1]. The Candida group with other

[*] Email: monia.elbour@instm.rnrt.tn

filamentous fungi, yeasts and yeast-like fungi were widely distributed in densities in water column [2] and microbiological quality surveys data for beach sands and waters, revealed mainly the presence of *C.albicans* with fecal coliforms [3]. This species was listed as the most Saccharomycete's present in European marine ecosystems [4].

According to several human health surveys data, *C.albicans* is listed as the most virulent species of Candida group and predominantes isolates found on oral mucosal layers, in vaginal infections and invasve blood stream infections [5, 6 and 7]. It's considered as an opportunistic fungus and a part of the normal microbial flora that colonizes mucocutaneous surfaces of oral cavity, gastrointestinal tract and vagina of many mammals, birds in terrestrial and aquattic environments [8]. The recent local or worldwide data pointed the incidence of *C.albicans* as human commensal fungus for more than 70% of healthy popultion which still ranged as the fourth leading cause of nosocomial blood stream infections with an attribuatable mortality rate of 37% - 44% in several immuno-compromised patients [9, 10]. The marine wildlife health data of [11] specified *C.albicans* as the most causative of fungal infections for the bottlenose dolphins (*Thursiops truncatus*) in south-eastern United States.

C.albicans is a polymorphic fungus that has the ability to switch between yeast and filamentous forms and still possess many putative virulence attributes contributing highly on its survival, fitness and persistence within the host and therefore can adopt both explorative and exploitative strategies with the formation of linear organs of aggregated hyphae to protect its translocation [1, 12, 13]. In a recent study [14], the authors shown that live filamentous *C.albicans* strains stimulate pro-inflammatory cytokine production in immune and non immune (epithelial) cells and this more invasive specie elicit higher levels of pro-inflammatory cytokines.

Further, *C.albicans* represents the main fungal species able to form biofilms and has the remarkable ability to grow in several distinct morphological forms: yeast, hyphae and pseudo-hyphae depending on environmental conditions [9] and therefore is less susceptible to antifungal agents compared to its planktonic counter parts. Thus, biofilm formation and its architectural development by the pathogen *C.albicans* still the main cause for large drug resistance of the fungi [15].

For all the previous reasons, effective alternatives still required to treat fungal infections, which are mainly caused by cells in biofilms [16]. More recent data [17], pointed the failure of antifungal therapy in immune-compromised patients related to the fungiastatic activity of azoles besides to the ability of *C.albicans* to form biofilms in most cases of candidiasis at both mucosal and systemic sites and signalled the lack of effective alternatives required for their treatment. Further, it has been well established that *C.albicans* biofilms are resistant to many antimicrobial agents including azoles, the most commonly class of antifungal drugs and therefore the efficacy of treatment for *C.albicans* infections, needs exploration of new antifungal strategies efficient against this fungi biofilms [18].

The recent exploring ocean studies, for new natural products highlighted large amounts of researches on natural products during the last decade of the 20th century and revealed the importance of marine organism as bio-producers of substances useful for the treatment of human diseases [19]. The inhibition of *C.albicans* extracellular enzyme activity by selected natural substances and their application in treatment of *C.albicans* infection was related to increase interest for pharmaceutical application against the most resistant pathogen fungi [20].

Here we summarize in two sections data available from our investigations and bibliographic studies about bio-activities against *C.albicans* from marine (i) macro-organisms and (ii) micro-organisms essentially from bacterial and fungal marine epibionts.

1. Candidiosis Bioactive Marine Macro-Organisms

The marine environment represents the main source for more than 20,000 inspirational natural products discovered over the past 50 years with mainly 9 approved drugs and 12 current clinical trial agents discovered, either as natural products or as molecules inspired from the natural product structure and with a significant degree, these have come from collections of phanerogams, algae and marine invertebrates largely obtained from shallow-water tropical ecosystems [21].

Within this large group of marine natural bioactive products, few were active against *C.albicans* (Table 1). The storage of biologically active secondary metabolites by marine invertebrates is frequently related to their ecological success, in spite of their exposition to predation, infestation by microbial pathogens, overgrowth, fouling and competition for space and nutrients and thus, marine sponges, ascidians, soft-bodied cnidaria and bryozoans are the main representative groups of the invertebrates which are chemically defended against predators [22].

Table 1. Bioactive marine macroorganisms against *C.albicans*

Taxon	Activities	Nature	References
Ascidian (Clavelina oblonga)	Positive	Polyketide	23
Polychetta (Arenicola marina)	Positive	Peptide (aremicins)	24
Gasteropod (Babylonia spirata)	Positive	Tissue extract	25
Sponges			
Dysidea arenaria	Positive	Terpene (sterol)	26
Hippospongia communis	Positive	Untenospongin B	27
I.variabilis	Positive	N.D*	27
Sp.dorigena	Positive	N.D*	27
G.cydonium	Positive	N.D*	27
H.offoculata	Positive	N.D*	27

*N.D: not determined.

Therefore, the results of screening for 349 crude extracts of Brazilian marine sponges, ascidians, bryozoans and octocorals against several antibiotic resistant micro-organisms, showed less than 10% species activities displayed against *C.albicans* [22]. Sponges (Porifera) are one of the richest sources of both biologically active secondary metabolites and chemical diversity nevertheless, present data reveal only six species with bioactive effect extracts against *C.albicans* (Table 1). Within the ascidian group, the two species *Clavelina oblonga* and *Didemunum sp* displayed inhibition against *C.albicans* and the bioactive polyketide substance has been successfully purified by [23]. Whereas for the Cnidaria and Bryozoan group the data of [22], related weak inhibition of an unidentified gorgonian to pathogen *C.albicans*.

The most recent study of [25] in southeast coast of India showed great medicinal value of muscle (tissues extracts) of the gasteropod (*Babylonia spiratat* Linnaeus, 1758 (Mollusca, Gasteropod) with high quality of antimicrobial compounds tested *in vitro* assays against *C.albicans*.

2. Candidiosis Bioactive Marine Micro-Organisms

In marine ecosystems, seaweeds and invertebrates microbial communities represent the true metabolic sources of most bioactive and valuable marine natural products accumulated within macro organism tissues and surfaces [28]. Several data revealed that, the number of novel compounds isolated from terrestrial microorganisms steadily decreased since late 1980s and marine environment represent the potential source for new bioactive antimicrobial mainly related to marine epibionts [29].

In previous study [30], local investigations on bacterial communities of some green, red and brown algae, revealed the high diversity and bacterial species associated with different genus of seaweeds and their antibiotic activities against several microbial pathogens mainly the fungi *Candida albicans* (Table 2).

Our studies highlighted the highest range of bacteria bioactive species related to the green algae species of *Ulva rigida*, *Ulva lactuca* and *Ulva intestinalis* against *C.albicans* and less bioactive epibionts from the red algae *Jania rubens* or the brown algae *Padina Pavonica* [31, 32]. Almost bioactive bacterial species identified belong to the Gamma proteobacteria group, secondly to the Alpha proteobacteria and less to the Bacteroides or Firmicutes groups. Within the Gamma proteobacteria we selected mainly species of *Pseudoalteromonas sp*, *Alteromonas sp* and *Pseudomonas sp* strong with bioactivities revealed both by cells and supernatant assays for all the bacteria species identified [30,33].

Other recent data specified a fungal extract of *Nocardia sp*. ALAA 2000, isolated from the marine red alga *Laurenica spectabilis* collected from the Red Sea coast in Egypt with high activity against pathogenic *Candida albicans* and other Gram+ and Gram- pathogen bacteria and fungi [34].

Within the invertebrate group mainly sponges harbour a rich diversity of microbial epibionts in their tissues which constitute in some case up to 40% of the sponge biomass, e.g. the Mediterranean sponge *Aplysina aerophoba* [35]. Considering that numerous natural products from marine invertebrates showed high structural similarities to metabolites of microbial origin, it suggest that microbial invertebrate epibionts are the true source of these metabolites or are intricately involved in their biosynthesis [36]. The available data signaled that almost sponge epibionts bioactive against *Candida albicans* were from bacteria group of Firmicutes or Gamma proteobacteria as specifically described in the Indian southern east coast sponges associated from what bacteria species of *Idiomarina baltica*, *Staphylococcus equorum*, *Bacillus sp*, *Pseudomonas sp* were isolated with bioactivity against *C.albicans* [37]. It's important to note that *Pseudomonas* and *Pseudoalteromonas* genera were the most bacterial bioactive species cited within available data [31, 32, 37 and 38].

Table 2. Bioactive marine microorganisms against *C.albicans*

Sources	Microorganism groups	Bioactive species	Extracts	References
Algae				
Ulva rigida	Gamma proteobacteria	*Acinetobacter johnsonii*	Cells	32
Ulva rigida	Gamma proteobacteria	*Alteromonas marina*	Cells	32
Ulva rigida	Gamma proteobacteria	*Alteromonas macleodii*	Cells	32
Ulva rigida	Bacteroides	*Bacteroidetes bacterium*	Cells	32
Ulva rigida	Firmicutes	*Bacillus sp.*	Cells	32
Ulva rigida	Alphaproteobacteria	*Dinoroseobacter shibae*	Cells	32
Ulva rigida	Firmicutes	*Enterococcus mundtii*	Cells	32
Ulva rigida	Alpha proteobacteria	*Labrenzia marina*	Cells	32
Ulva rigida	Alpha proteobacteria	*Nereida ignava*	Cells	32
Ulva rigida	Alpha proteobacteria	*Octadecabacter sp.*	Cells	32
Ulva rigida	Gamma proteobacteria	*Pseudoalteromonas sp*	Cells	32
Ulva rigida	Gamma proteobacteria	*Psychroserpens mesophilus*	Cells	32
Ulva rigida	Alpha proteobacteria	*Rhodobacteraceae bacterium*	Cells	32
Ulva rigida	Alpha proteobacteria	*Ruegeria sp.*	Cells	32
Ulva rigida	Bacteroides	*Salegentibacter sp.*	Cells	32
Ulva rigida	Firmicutes	*Staphylococcus arlettae*	Cells	32
Ulva lactuca	Gamma proteobacteria	*Pseudoalteromonas aurantia*	Cells	33
Ulva rigida et Ulva intestinalis	Alpha proteobacteria	*Stappia sp.*	Cells	32
Jania rubens	Bacteroides	*Aquimarina sp.*	Cells	31
Jania rubens	Firmicutes	*Bacillus pumilus*	Cells	31
Jania rubens	Alpha proteobacteria	*Paracoccus sp.*	Cells	31
Jania rubens	Gamma proteobacteria	*Pseudoalteromonas sp*	Cells	31
Jania rubens	Gamma proteobacteria	*Pseudomonas sp*	Cells	31
Dictyota bartaryresiana	Actinobacteria	*Actinobacteria spp*	Cells	39
Digenaea sp	Gamma proteobacteria	*Pseudoalteromonas sp*	Cells	38
Padina pavonica	Firmicutes	*Bacillus pumilus*	Cells	32
Padina pavonica	Gamma proteobacteria	*Pseudoalteromonas sp*	Cells	32
Padina pavonica	Gamma proteobacteria	*Pseudomonas sp*	Cells	32
Diginea sp	Gamma proteobacteria	*Pseudomonas sp*	Cells	38
Invertebrates				
Sponges				
Echinodictyums sp		*Idiomarina baltica*	Cells	37
Spongia sp	Firmicutes	*Staphylococcus equorum*	Cells	37
Sigmadocia fibulatus	Firmicutes	*Bacillus sp*	Cells	37

Table 2. (Continued)

Sources	Microorganism groups	Bioactive species	Extracts	References
Sigmadocia fibulatus	Gamma proteobacteria	*Pseudomonas sp*	Cells	37
Bivalves				
Marine ark shell (Anadara broughtoni)	Firmicutes	*Bacillus pumilus*	Cells	28
Marine ark shell (Anadara broughtoni)	Firmicutes	*Paemobacillus polymyxa*	Cells	28
Marine ark shell (Anadara broughtoni)		*Sphingomonas asaccharolyticus*	Cells	28
Water or sediment				
Marine water		*Streptomyces sp*	Cell metabolite	29
Marine mud	Gamma proteobacteria	*Pseudoalteromonas issachenkonii*	Supernatant	40
Marine mud		*Patero.luteoviolacea*	Cells	40
Lakes mats	Beta proteobacteria	*Janthinobacterium lividum*	Cells	41
Lakes mats	Beta proteobacteria	*Hydrogenophaga palleronii*	Cells	41
Saline lakes	Fungi	*Aspergillus clavatus*	novel substance (n.i)	43
Marine mud	Fungi	*Massarina sp*	Crude	43
Marine mud	Yeast	*Marakia frigida*	Killer toxins	46
Floating scrap	Fungi	*Ascophyta sp*	Crude	44

Further, a putative new genus related to *Rubrobacter* of the actinomycete group was isolated from marine sponges in Egypt and Croatia and tested with anti-infective activities against *Candida albicans* and other bacterial pathogens and human parasites [39]. These data show a high diversity of microbial epibionts related with marine sponges and highlight their bioactive potential and production of anti-infective agents. From the marine bivalve group, a recent study highlight incidence of metabolites extracts of the ark shell *Anadara broughtoni* inhabiting the Sea of Japan [28]. The bivalve was assessed for its microbial diversity and was shown to harbour several bacterial epibionts (from Firmicutes group, Table 2) responsible of potential bioactivities on *C.albicans* and other pathogens assessed *in vitro* by diffusion tests [28]. Besides organisms, the marine sediments have been explored for bioactive microbial species and recent data described several bioactive bacterial and fungal species [40, 41], nevertheless few species displayed activities against *C.albicans* (Table 2). Thus, two species of Beta proteobacteria (*Janthinobacterium lividum* and *Hydrogenophaga palleronii*) were isolated from benthic antarctic lakes mats as a source of new bioactive metabolites [42] whereas another study [39] described a novel copper resistant and antimicrobial Streptomyces isolated from the Bay of Bengal in India positively tested *in vitro* assays against *C.albicans* and [29], described similar antifungal activities of polyketide metabolite extracted from marine *Streptomyces sp* AP123 against *C.albicans* and several other pathogens.

Besides bacteria, fungal epibionts were isolated mainly from marine sediments with high bioactivities against *C. albicans* (Table 2). Therefore, toxicity of *C.albicans* to more than 17 benthic mats fungi was described by [44] and mostly related to the genus *Thelebolis, Penicelluim, Aspergillus, Curvulana, Geomycis* and *Cladosporium*. Thus, two bis-anthraquinones (rugulosin and skyrin) were purified and characterized from the specie *Penicellium chrysogenum* (IWW1053) isolated from saline Highway lake in India and less bioactive compound was identified from the specie *Aspergillus clavatus* (IWW447).

Another marine-derived fungus, *Ascochyta sp*. NGB4, was isolated from a floating scrap of festering rope at a fishing port in Japan and the chemical investigation of this strain yielded a new spirodioxynaphthalene metabolite, named ascochytatin which exhibited relatively strong and specific activity against Gram+ bacteria and *C. albicans* [45]. Within yeast group few studies [46, 47] screened antimicrobial active metabolites active against *C.albicans*, isolated from shore coast in Iran and sea sediments in the Antarctica and the cold active "killer toxin" (MW = 55,6Kda) from the psychrotolerant yeast (*Mrakia frigida*) was purified and characterized. The "Killer toxins" are extracellular toxins produced by certain yeast species or strains which kill sensitive yeasts, but not the producer strain [47]. Nevertheless the large antimicrobial spectrum described for a wide range of marine microbial epibionts, great efforts remain to be solved for further medicinal specific substances against *C. albicans* which remain less sensitive to major antimicrobial extracts assessed as highlighted by several studies [41, 43]. The recent study [48] focusing on the diversity of surface marine bacteria revealed no specific activity for all the bioactive isolates against *C.albicans*.

Conclusion

Biological activities of marine organisms against the most causative fungal infections *C.albicans* have been reviewed in this chapter. Marine microbial communities free-living (in sediment or column water) or associated to algae, phanerogams or invertebrates represent the high relevant sources of metabolites with clinical utility and applications against *C.albicans* eventhough lower sensitivity observed for this species to large amount of marine metabolites compared to several antibioresistant other pathogen bacteria and fungi. The available data revealed that the major part of marine antimicrobial metabolites were not completely investigated and remain to be well characterized taking in account variations in environment marine ecosystems to setup effective alternatives which still required to treat fungal infections taking in account hich tech innovation for multidisciplinary exploration of the marine metabolites for their pharmaceutical applications against anbioresistant pathogens.

References

[1] Gadd G.M. 2007. Geomycology: biogeochemical transformations of rocks, minerals, metals and radionuclides by fungi, bioweathering and bioremediation. *Mycological Research*, 111, 3-49.

[2] Kwaswieska K. 1988.Horizontal distribution and diversity of yeasts and filamentous fungi in Lake St Clair. *Journal of Great Lakes Research*, 14-4, 438-443.

[3] El Manama A.A, Fahd M.I, Afifi S., AbdAllah S., Bahr S. 2005. Microbiological beach sand quality in Gaza strip in comparison to seawater quality. *Environmental Reaserch,* 99, 1-10.

[4] Landy E.T & Jones J. 2006. What is the fungal diversity of marine ecosystems in Europe? *Mycologist,* 20: 15-21.

[5] Arendrup M.C, Fursted K., Gahrn-Hansen B., Schønheyder H.C., Knudsen J.D., Jensen I.M. 2005. Semi national surveillance of furgenia in Denmark, notably high rates of reduced azole susceptibility. *Journal of Clinical Microbiology*, 43: 4434-40.

[6] Pfaller M.A & Diekena D.J. 2007. Epidemiology of invasive candidiasis: a persistent public health problem. *Clinical Microbiological Reviews*, 20: 133-63.

[7] Samaranayake L & Keurg P., Leung W., Jin I. 2009. Oral mucosal fungal infections. *Periodontol* 2000. 49: 39-59.

[8] Buluc M., Atagl U.H., Dogave D., Ergun H., Gurdal H., Erdenli E., Denirel-Yilmaz E. 2005. Effect of *C.albicans* septicemia on the cardiovascular function of rabbit. *International Immunopharmacology*, 5: 893-901.

[9] Hau T.L, Cannon R.D, Villas-Bôas G. 2011.The metabolic basis of *Candida albicans* morphogenesis and quorum sensing. *Fungal Genetics and Biology*, 48: 747-763.

[10] Saghrouni F., Bouguiza I., Ben AbdelJellil J., Yacoub A., Khammari I., FathAllah A., Mtiraoui A., Ben Said M. 2011. Epidemiological trends in invasive candidiasis: results from a 15 years study in Sousse region, Tunisia. *Journal de Mycologie Médicale,* 21: 123-129.

[11] Morris P.J., Johnson W.R., Pisani J., Bossart G.D., Adams J., Reif J.S., Fair P.A. 2011. Isolation of culturable micro-organisms from free-ranging bottlenose dolphins (*Tursiops truncatus*) from Southeastern United States. *Veterinarian Microbiology*, 148: 440-447.

[12] Frade J.P., Arthington-Skaggs B.A. 2011.Effect of serum and surface characteristics on *C.albicans* biofilm formation. *Mycoses,* 54: e154-e162.

[13] Naglik J.R., Moyers D.L., Wächtler B., Benhard H. 2011.*Candida albicans* interactions with epithelial cels and mucosal immunity. *Microbes and Infections*, 13: 963-976.

[14] Whiley R.A., Crucheley A.T., Gore C., Pavli E.H. 2012.*C.albicans* strain dependent modulation of pro-inflammatory cytokine release by *in vitro* oral and vaginal mucosal models, *Cytokine* 57: 89-97.

[15] Chandra J. 2001a. Biofilm formation by the fungal pathogen *C.albicans*: development, architecture and drug resistance. *Journal of Bacteriology*, 183: 5385-5394.

[16] Gonzales F.P., Marsh T. 2012.Photodynamic inactivation for controlling *C.albicans* infections. *Fungal Biology*, 116: 1-10.

[17] Arana D.M., Nombela C., Pla J. 2010.Fluconazole at subinhibitory conventrations induces the oxidative and nitrosative responses genes TRR1, GRE2 and YHB1 and enhances the resistance of *C.albicans* to phagocytes. *Journal of Antimicrobial Chemotherapy,* 65: 54-62.

[18] Yu O., Ding X., Xu N., Cheng X., Quian K., Zhang B.2013. *In vitro* activity of Nerapamil alone and in combination with fluconazole on tunicamycin against biofilms. *International Journal od Antimicrobial Agents*, 41: 179-182.

[19] Imhoff JF., Labes A., Wiese, J.2011. Bio-mining the microbial treasures of the ocean: new natural products. *Biotechnological Advances*, 29: 468-482.

[20] Yordanov M. 2008.Inhibition of *C.albicans* extra-cellular enzyme activity by selected natural substances and their applications in *Candida* infection. *Canadian Journal of Microbiology*, 54: 435-440.

[21] Gerwick K.W.H., Fenner A.M.2013.Drug discovery from marine microbes. *Microbial Ecology,* 63: 800-806.

[22] Seleghim M.H.R., Lira S.P., Kossuga M.R., Batista T., Berlinck R.G.S., Hajdu E., Muricy G., Da Rocha M.R., Do Nascimento G.F., Silva M., Pimenta E.F., Thiemann O.T., Oliva G., Cavalcanti B.C., Pessoa C., De Moraes A., Galetti F.S.C., Silva S.C., De Souza A., Peixinho S.2007.Antibiotic, cytotoxic and enzyme inhibitory activity of crude extracts from Brazilian marine invertebrates. *Brazilian Journal of Pharmacognosy*, 17(3): 287-318.

[23] Kossuga M.H., McMillan J.B., Rogers E.W., Molinski J.F., Nacimento G.G., Rocha R.M., Berlinck R.G. 2004. (2S, 3R)-2-aminododecan-3-ol a new antifungal agent from the ascidian *Clavelina oblonga*. *Journal of Natural Products*, 67: 1879-1881.

[24] Ovchinnikova T.V., Aleshina G.M., Balandin S.V., Krasnosdembskaya A.D.,Markelov M.L., Frolova E.I., Leonova Y.F., Tagaev A.A., KrasnodembskyE.G., Kokryakov V.N.2004.Purification and primary structure of two isoforms of arenicin, a novel antimicrobial peptide from marine polychaeta Arenicola marina. *FEBS Letters*. 577, 209–214.

[25] Periyasamy N., Srinivasan M., Balakrishnan S.2012. Antimicrobial activities of the tissue extracts of *Babylonia spirata* Linnaeus, 1758 (Mollusca: Gastropoda) from Thazhanguda, southeast coast of *India Asian Pacific Journal of Tropical Biomedicine*, 2012: 36-40.

[26] Jacob M.R., Hossain C.F., Mohammed K.A., Smillie T.J., Clark A.M., Walker L.A., Nagle D.G., 2003. Reversal of fluconazole resistance in multidrug efflux-resistant fungi by the Dysidea arenaria sponge sterol 9alpha, 11alpha-epoxycholest-7-ene-3beta, 5alpha,6alpha,19-tetrol 6-acetate. *Journal of Natural Product*, 66: 1618–1622.

[27] Rifai S., Fassouane A., Kijjoa A., Van Soest R., 2004.Antimicrobial activity of untenospongin B, a metabolite from the marine sponge Hippospongia communis collected from the Atlantic coast of Morocco. *Marine Drugs,* 2: 147–153.

[28] Romanenko L.A., Uchino M., Kalinoskaya N.I., Mikhailov V.V.2008. Isolation, phylogenetic analysis and screening of marine mollusc – associated bacteria for antimicrobial, hemolytic and surfaces activities. *Microbial Reaserch*, 163: 633-644.

[29] Arasu M.V., Duraipandiyan V., Ignacimuthu S. 2013.Antibacterial and antifungal activities of polyketide metabolite from marine *Streptomyces sp.* AP123 and its cytotoxic effect. *Chemosphere.* 90: 479-487.

[30] El Bour M., Ismail-BenAli A., Ktari L. Microbiology Book Series "microbial pathogens and strategies for combating them: Science, *Technology and Education.* 2013. In press.

[31] Ismail-Ben Ali A.; El Bour M.; Ktari L.; Bolhuis H.; Ahmed M.; Boudabbous A.; Stal L.J. 2011. *Jania rubens*-associated bacteria: molecular identification and antimicrobial activity. *Journal of Applied Phycology, DOI10.1007/s10811-011*, 9758-0.

[32] Ismail-Ben Ali A., El Bour M., Ktari L., Bolhuis H., Ahmed M., Boudabous A., Stal L.J. 2012. Comparative study of epiphytic bacteria associated with two algae from Cap Zebib (Northern Tunisia). *TJASSST-11 proceedings*.

[33] Bowman J.P.2007.Bioactive compound synthetic capacity and ecological significance of marine bacterial genus *Pseudoalteromonas*. *Marine Drugs,* 5-4: 220-41.

[34] Hughes C.C., Prieto-Davo A., Jensen P.R., Fenical, W.2008.The marinopyrroles, antibiotics of an unprecedented structure class from a marine *Streptomyces sp*. *Organic Letters,* 10: 629–631.

[35] Friedrich A.B., Merkert H., Fendert T., Hacker J., Proksh P., Hentschel U.1999. Microbial diversity in the marine sponge *Aplysina cavernicula* (formerly *verongia cavernicola*) analyzed by fluorescence in situ hybridization (FISH). *Marine Biology,* 134: 461-470.

[36] Proksch P., Ebel R., Edrada R.A., Riebe F., Liu H., Diesel, A.2008. Sponge-associated fungi and their bioactive compounds: the Suberites case. *Bot Mar*, 51: 209–218.

[37] Anaud T.R., Bhat A.W., Shouche Y.S., Roy U., Siddhartha P.S.2006. Antimicrobial activity of marine bacteria associated with spongesfrom waters off the coast of South East India. *Microbiological Research*, 161: 252-262.

[38] Dhahiya R., and Hemendra G.2011.Toward the Synthesis and Biological Screening of a Cyclotetrapeptide from Marine Bacteria. *Marine Drugs*, 9: 71-81.

[39] Ramadan A., Pimentel-Elardo S.M., Hanora A., Radwan M., Abou-El-Ela S.H., Ahmed S., Hentschel U.2010. *Marine Drugs*, 8: 399-412.

[40] Kalinovskaya N.I., Ivanova E.P., Alexeeva Y.Y., Gorshkova N.M., Kuznetsova T.A., Dmitrenok S.K., Nicolau D.V.2004.Low-Molecular-Weight, Biologically Active Compounds from Marine *Pseudoalteromonas* species. *Current Microbiology*, 48: 441–446.

[41] Rojas J.L., Martin J., Torno J.R., Vicente F., Gerrillond O.2009.bacterial diversity from benthic mats of antarctic lakes as a source of new bioactive metabolites. *Marine Genomics,* 2: 33-41.

[42] Yadav A.K., Kumar R., Saikia R., Bora T.C., Arora D.K.2009.Novel copper resistant and antimicrobial Streptomyces isolated from Bay of Bengal, India. *Journal de Mycologie Médicale,* 19: 234-240.

[43] Brumati M., Rojas J.L., Sponga F., Ciciliato I., Losi D., Göttlich E., DeHoog S., Genilloud O., Marinelli F.2009.Diversity and pharmaceutical screening of fungi from benthic mats of antactic lakes. *Marine Genomics*, 2: 43-50.

[44] Kanoh K., Okada A., Adachi K., Imagawa H., Nishizawa M., Matsuda S.2008. Ascochytatin, a novel bioactive spirodioxynaphthalene metabolite produced by the marine-derived fungus, Ascochyta sp. NGB4. *J. Antibiot., 61*: 142–148.

[45] Mehrvar M., Sardari S.2011.Screening of antimicrobial membrane active metabolites of soil microfungi by using chromatic phospholipid /polydiactylene vesicles. *Journal de Mycologie Médicale*, 21: 188-197.

[46] Liu G.L., Wang K., Hua M.X., Buzdar M.A., Chi Z.M.2012. Purification and characterization of the cold –active killer toxin from the psychotolerant yeast Mrakia frigida isolated from sea sediments in Antarctica. *Process Biochemistry*, 47: 822-827.

[47] Wilson G.S., Raftos D.A., Corrigan S.L., Nair S.V.2009.Diversity and antimicrobial activities of surface –attached marine bacteria from Sydney Harbour, Australia. *Microbiological Research*, 165: 300-311.

[48] Mayer AMS, Rodriguez A.D., Berlink R.G.S., Berlink R.G.S., Hamann M.T.2007.Marine pharmacology in 2003-4: marine compounds with anthelminthic antibacterial, anticoagulant, antifungal anti-inflammatory , antimalarial, antiplatelet, antiprotozoal antituberculosis and antiviral activities affecting the cardiovascular, immune and nervous systems and other miscellaneous mechanisms of action. *Comparative Biochemistry and Physiology* Part C, 145: 553-581.

In: Candida *albicans*: Symptoms, Causes and Treatment Options ISBN: 978-1-62808-882-3
Editors: Leon A. Dietrich and Tim S. Friedmann

Chapter X

Polyenes, Azoles and Echinocandins for Treating Infections Caused by *Candida albicans* and Other *Candida* Species

Tzi Bun Ng**, *Jack Ho Wong** and *Charlene Cheuk Wing Ng
School of Biomedical Sciences,Faculty of Medicine,
The Chinese University of Hong Kong, New Territories,
Hong Kong, China

Abstract

Invasive fungal infection (IFI) is a serious problem since it is difficult to diagnose early and mortality is high. A variety of approaches are adopted for the therapy and management of IFI including prophylactic, empiric, preemptive, and directed strategies. Lipid formulations of amphotericin B (colloidal dispersion, lipid complex and liposomal) are better tolerated than amphotericin B deoxycholate and are equally effective. The lipid formulations have usually been used as second-line therapy in patients with refractory invasive candidiasis. Azole drugs are frequently used in cost-effective antifungal prophylaxis of patients with immunodeficiency and cancer that increase the susceptibility to invasive fungal infection. Fluconazole is the best known example. Echinocandins have desirable characteristics that render make them useful for treating Candida infections. Antibodies or their engineered derivatives directed against cell-wall polysaccharides and glycopeptides, and some protein epitopes of *Candida albicans* are seemingly a novel approach for prophylaxis against Candida infection and merit further in-depth studies.

Keywords: Antifungal prophylaxis, amphotericin, azoles, echinocandins

* Email addresses of corresponding author : b021770@mailserv.cuhk.edu.hk (TBNg), jack1993@yahoo.com (JH Wong), fax: 852 26035123, phone: 852 39436872.

Introduction

Invasive fungal infection (IFI) is a problem hard to tackle due to the difficulties in making an early diagnosis and high mortality. Different approaches are adopted for the treatment and management of IFI comprising prophylactic, empiric, preemptive, and directed strategies. It is crucial to make an early intervention inasmuch as the probability of treating an infection diminishes as the infection progresses. Some circumstances elevate the risk of IFI. Results of randomized, controlled clinical investigations have revealed the advantages of antifungal prophylaxis (Cornely et al., 2011). A review of the experience of two sizeable successive surveillance programs, the SENTRY Antimicrobial Surveillance Program (2006-2010) and the Centers for Disease Control and Prevention population-based surveillance (2008-2010), disclosed the broad emergence of coresistance to both azole drugs and echinocandins in clinical isolates of *Candida. glabrata* over time (Pfaller et al., 2012). The purpose of the present review article is to gather published evidence pertaining to the efficacy of antifungal prophylaxis in preventing IFI. The antifungal drugs covered include polyenes, azoles and echinocandins.

1. Polyenes

Amphotericin B deoxycholate has been used as the standard treatment for invasive fungal infections for many years. However, it is poorly tolerated and there are side effects such as acute infusion-related reactions and nephrotoxicity. Lipid formulations of amphotericin B (colloidal dispersion, lipid complex and liposomal) are better tolerated than amphotericin B deoxycholate and are equally effective. The lipid formulations have usually been used as second-line therapy in patients with refractory invasive candidiasis due to the high costs and availability of azoles and echinocandins for alternative antifungal therapy (Méan et al., 2008). Intravenous amphotericin were commonly administered to infants with very low birth weight (Wilkerson et al., 2010).

2. Azoles

(a) Fluconazole

Intravenous fluconazole was administered to infants with very low birth weight (Wilkerson et al., 2010).The fluconazole prophylaxis regimen inhibited invasive Candida infection in infants with extremely low birth weight (Bhat et al., 2011) without long-term deleterious effects on brain development and quality of life (Kaufman et al., 2011). Fluconazole prophylaxis may be of some benfit to critically ill neonates at high risk with risk factors such as therapy with broad-spectrum antibiotics, central venous access, or units with high incidence of invasive fungal infection (Reed et al., 2010).

Fluconazole has been a standard option for antifungal prophylaxis in children with cancer (Giacchino et al., 2010). However, there is no consensus on the dosage of voriconazole and posaconazole for these patients (Dvorak et al., 2010).

Fluconazole prophylaxis is justified in high-risk liver transplant recipients but not in low-risk patients (San-Juan et al., 2011).In HIV-positive women with vulvovaginal candidiasis, fluconazole was effective for prevention (Ray et al., 2011).

(b) Itraconazole

Itraconazole had higher efficacy than fluconazole in reducing fungal infections and invasive fungal infections in neutropenic patients with hematological malignancies (Wang et al., 2010).The drug inhibited non-invasive and invasive candidiases in immunosuppressed patients receiving moderate or high doses of corticosteroids (Iriyama et al., 2011).

(c) Posaconazole

Posaconazole, which shows broad-spectrum activity against a diversity of filamentous fungi and yeasts, is administered orally for the treatment of oropharyngeal candidiasis and prophylaxis of invasive fungal infections in immunosuppressed hosts. It is well tolerated by patients. However, due to gastrointestinal absorption problems its efficacy in treating deep-seated infections is attenuated (Ianas et al., 2010).

Posaconazole exhibited higher prophylactic efficacy than standard azoles in neutropenic patients with acute myelogenous leukaemia or myelodysplastic syndromes and at risk of invasive fungal infection (Lazzaro, 2010). Patients with acute lympoblastic leukemia receiving intensified induction phase treatment and given a prophylactic dose of posaconazole experienced side effects that were, however, not life-threatening (Illmer et al., 2011).

Posaconazole treatment of hematopoietic stem-cell transplantation recipients led to a reduced incidence of invasive fungal infections, more life-years gained and higher invasive fungal infection-related cost/patient than fluconazole treatment (de la Cámara et al., 2010)

Posaconazole prevented invasive fungal infections in chemotherapy-induced neutropenic patients with acute myelogenous leukaemia or myelodysplastic syndromes. Posaconazole and fluconazole were equally effective on patients with graft-versus-host disease who received intensive immunosuppressive therapy following hematopoietic stem cell transplantation. Mortality due to invasive fungal infection declined after posaconazole prophylaxis (Lyseng-Williamson, 2011).

(d) Voriconazole

Recurrence of prior invasive fungal infection may take place after stem cell transplantation. Nevertheless, secondary prophylaxis may reduce the disease burden and enhance survival with. A prospective, open-label, multicenter trial was executed, to test voriconazole (4 mg/kg/12 h intravenously or 200 mg/12 h orally) as a secondary antifungal prophylactic agent in allogeneic stem cell transplant recipients with previous confirmed or probable invasive fungal infection. Therapy commenced 48 h or more after conditioning chemotherapy was over. Patients were followed for one year, with incidence of proven/probable invasive fungal infection as the primary end-point. Forty-five patients were enrolled, 41 of whom suffered from acute leukemia. Eleven patients (24%) died within the first year following transplantation, but only one death was attributed to systemic fungal disease. There were three invasive fungal infections after transplantation. The 1-year cumulative incidence of invasive fungal disease was 6.7±3.6%, considerably lower than the relapse rate reported in historical controls. The safety and effectiveness of voriconazole seemed to be satisfactory (Cordonnier et al., 2010).

3. Echinocandins

The efficacy and safety of caspofungin were similar to standard policy prophylactic regimens IFI (Cattaneo et al., 2011).

Doses of micafungin in adult (100 mg/day, 150 mg/day) and in pediatric (3 mg/kg/day) hematopoietic stem cell transplant recipients, after treatment with vinca alkaloids, have been found to be effective and safe. Micafungin elicits activity against Candida, displays favorable pharmacokinetic profile and is devoid of drug interactions. The optimal and cost-effective prophylactic dose and alternatives to daily intravenous administration, await elucidation (Salavert and Jarque, 2011).

Echinocandins (caspofungin, micafungin and anidulafungin) inhibit an enzyme pivotal to fungal cell wall integrity and are employed for the treatment of candidemia and invasive candidiasis in moderately to severely ill patients. The drugs demonstrate good antimicrobial potency and pharmacological properties (de la Cámara et al., 2010).

Caspofungin is cost-effective for the treatment of invasive candidiasis and also empirical treatment of suspected infections. Micafungin is an alternative to amphotericin B for prophylaxis in haematopoietic stem cell transplant patients and is cost-effective in prophylaxis even in the presence of fluconazole resistance. Anidulafungin is also cost-effective in a pharmacoeconomic model. Caspofungin, micafungin, and nidulafungin do not cost more than other treatment option (Wilke, 2011). They are well tolerated by pediatric cancer patients, but only the intravenous form is available.

In a randomized, double-blind investigation using patients with invasive candidiasis , anidulafungin (100 mg/day subsequent to a 200 mg dose) was superior to fluconazole (400 mg/day subsequent to a 800 mg loading dose), but noninferiority was reported after removal of the center that enrolled the largest number of patients. A randomized, double-blind study compared micafungin (100 or 150 mg/day) and caspofungin (70 mg loading dose and then 50 mg/day) in 595 adult patients with candidemia or invasive candidiasis noninferior efficacy of micafungin compared with that of caspofungin and similar safety profiles for the two compounds reported (Scott et al., 2012).

In critically ill patients, invasive candidiasis accounts for high morbidity and mortality. Antifungal therapy is implemented in critically ill patients with risk for candidemia (prophylaxis). Systemic antifungal therapy is also instituted in patients at increased risk for invasive candidiasis (preemptive therapy), or in patients with unresolving sepsis in spite of appropriate management (empirical therapy). Recently, better identification of patients who may benefit from echinocandin or polyene therapy, and others who are treatable by azole derivatives, can be achieved. However, prospective trials are still needed to better identify appropriate therapy for patients at risk for, or with, confirmed invasive Candida infections (Echeverria et al., 2011)

There is a dearth of information pertaining to clinical applications of antibodies in immunoprophylaxis of Candida infections although the results of several investigations look encouraging. Antibodies or their engineered derivatives directed against cell-wall polysaccharides and glycopeptides, and some protein epitopes of *Candida albicans* exhibit a protective action against invasive candidiasis. A human recombinant monoclonal antibody that inhibits heat shock protein 90, designated as Mycograb, has been employed in combination therapy with lipid-associated amphotericin B, in patients with invasive candidiasis. The antifungal anti-beta-glucan antibodies induced by the glycoconjugate vaccine composed of a beta-glucan polysaccharide conjugated with the diphtheria toxoid CRM 197, are also available Cabezas et al., 2010).

Postsurgical patients in intensive care units have a heightened risk of bloodstream Candida infections. Antifungal prophylaxis brings economic benefit, but its utility and cost-benefits should be assessed since available information is not adequate to lead to general recommendations (Cataldo and Petrosillo, 2010).

Conclusion

This article reviews drugs used in prophylaxis of invasive candida infections which may lead to high mortality. Fluconazole prophylaxis is administered to infants with very low and extremely low birth weights, pediatric patients with heart disease, preterm neonates, adult cancer patients with neutropenia, HIV-infected patients, and HIV-positive women with vulvovaginal candidiasis. To pediatric cancer patients, liposomal amphotericin B, fluconazole and micafungin are given. Itraconazole is administered to pediatric autologous allogeneic hematopoietic stem cell transplantation recipients and immunosuppressed patients treated with moderate or high doses of corticosteroids. To adult patients with hematologic malignancy, posaconazole, fluconazole voriconazole and caspofungin are given. Posaconazole is administered to allogeneic blood and marrow transplantation recipients. Patients with invasive fusariosis are treated with itraconazole. Hematopoietic stem-cell transplantation (alloHCT) recipients are treated with itraconazole, voriconazole, posaconazole, micafungin, caspofungin and amphotericin B. Heart transplant recipients receive itraconazole or inhaled amphotericin. Lung transplant recipients are treated with voriconazole, inhaled amphotericin B, echinocandins, and posaconazole. Anidulafungin is indicated to HIV-seropositive liver transplant recipients. Candidemia and invasive candidiasis are treated with echinocandins (caspofungin, micafungin and anidulafungin) and posaconazole. Systemic mycoses are treated with fluconazole, voriconazole, itraconazole and posaconazole. Antifungal prophylaxis is beneficial and reduces mortality in patients at high risk of invasive fungal infection.

Invasive candidiasis is the most frequent invasive mycosis in critically ill patients. Changing epidemiology with increased non-*albicans Candida* spp., nonspecific risk factors and clinical presentation, and late diagnosis with culture-based methods are major challenges in the management of invasive candidiasis. Preventive strategies targeting patients with a high-risk profile, development of new noninvasive diagnostic tools that allow early diagnosis and therapy, and extension of the therapeutic armamentarium with new agents are encouraging recent advances that may enable us to overcome *Candida* infections.

Azole drugs are the drugs most often used in cost-effective antifungal prophylaxis of patients with conditions such as immunodeficiency and cancer that render them highly susceptible to invasive fungal infection. Fluconazole is the most outstanding example. However, there are many azoles with different pharmacological characteristics that the physician can choose from. Echinocandins have favorable characteristics that make them useful for treating Candida infections. Antibodies or their engineered derivatives directed against cell-wall polysaccharides and glycopeptides, and some protein epitopes of *Candida albicans* appear to be a promising novel approach for prophylaxis against Candida infection and deserve further in-depth investigations. Discovery of more drugs with different pharmacological characteristics and mechanisms of action would certainly augment the armamentarium against pathogenic fungi that can cause high mortality.

The emerging fungal resistance to currently available antifungals for coping with fungal infections warants a hunt for new therapeutics. The incidence of infections by pathogenic Candida species rises because of the use of invasive procedures and immunosuppressive drugs for organ transplants and frequent administration of broad-spectrum antibiotics. *C. albicans* is implicated in the bulk of candidiasis (Beck-Sague and Jarvis, 1993) which constitutes the fourth most frequent nosocomial infection involving both mucosal and deep tissues, with mortality that may rise above 40%. *C. albicans* forms biofilms on mucosal surfaces and implanted medical devices, such as intravenous catheters. Biofilms, which might be responsible for a considerable percentage of infections in which cells adhere to a surface and embed in a matrix of extracellular polymeric substances secreted by these cells, exist in central venous catheters (Kim and Sudbery, 2011) and are recalcitrant to exixting antifungals. Thus new antifungal agents are badly needed, in particular those that have efficacy against Candida biofilms (Mandal et al., 2011).

C. albicans biofilms exhibit increased resistance to antifungal agents such as fluconazole and amphotericin B and host immune defenses (Chandra et al., 2001). Human cathelicidin(Benincasa et al., 2006; Wong and Ng, 2011)and lactoferrin and its peptide derivatives (Kobayashi et al., 2011; Bolscher et al., 2012) manifest activity against *C. albicans* including drug-resistant strains. They represent new peptide/protein candidates for antifungal prophylaxis.

Acknowledgments

The award of a research grant (Research Funds for the Control of Infectious Diseases, project reference no. 10090812) by Food and Health Bureau, the Government of Hong Kong Special Administrative Region, is gratefully acknowledged.

References

Beck-Sague, CM, Jarvis, WR. National nosecomial infections surveillance system. Secular trends in the epidemiology of nosocomial fungal infections in the United states 1980-1990. *J Infect Dis* 1993;167:1247-1251.

Benincasa M, Scocchi M, Pacor S, et al. Fungicidal activity of five cathelicidin peptides against clinically isolated yeasts. *J Antimicrob Chemother* 2006;58:950-959.

Bhat V, Fojas M, Saslow JG, et al. Twice-weekly fluconazole prophylaxis in premature infants: association with cholestasis. *Pediatr Int* 2011;53:475-9.

Bolscher J, Nazmi K, van Marle J, et al. Chimerization of lactoferricin and lactoferrampin peptides strongly potentiates the killing activity against *Candida albicans. Biochem Cell Biol* 2012 [Epub ahead of print]

Cabezas J, Albaina O, Montañez D, et al. Potential of anti-Candida antibodies in immunoprophylaxis. *Immunotherapy* 2010;2:171-83.

Cataldo MA, Petrosillo N. Economic considerations of antifungal prophylaxis in patients undergoing surgical procedures. *Ther Clin Risk Manag* 2011;7:13-20.

Cattaneo C, Monte S, Algarotti A, et al. Itraconazole vs fluconazole as a primary prophylaxis for fungal infections in HIV-infected patients in Thailand. *Curr HIV Res* 2011;9:334-8.

Chandra J, Mukherjee PK, Leidich SD, et al. Antifungal resistance of candidal biofilms formed on denture acrylic *in vitro*. *J Dent Res* 2001;80:903-908.

Cornely OA, Aversa F, Cook P, et al. Evaluating the role of prophylaxis in the management of invasive fungal infections in patients with hematologic malignancy. *Eur J Haematol* 2011;87:289-301.

de la Cámara R, Jarque I, Sanz MA, et al. Economic evaluation of posaconazole vs fluconazole in the prevention of invasive fungal infections in patients with GVHD following haematopoietic SCT. *Bone Marrow Transplant* 2010;45:925-32.

Dvorak CC, Fisher BT, Sung L, et al. Antifungal prophylaxis in pediatric hematology/oncology: New choices & new data. *Pediatr Blood Cancer* 2011;[Epub ahead of print]

Echeverria PM, Kett DH, Azoulay E. Candida prophylaxis and therapy in the ICU. *Semin Respir Crit Care Med* 2011;32:159-73.

Giacchino M, Milano GM, Carraro F, et al. Current evidence of antifungal prophylaxis and therapy in pediatric patients. *Pediatr Rep* 2011;3:e6.

Ianas V, Matthias KR, Klotz SA. Role of posaconazole in the treatment of oropharyngeal candidiasis. *Infect Drug Resist* 2010;3:45-51.

Illmer T, Babatz J, Pursche S, et al. Posaconazole prophylaxis during induction therapy of patients with acute lymphoblastic leukaemia. *Mycoses* 2011;54:e143-7.

Iriyama N, Matsukawa Y, Miura K, et al. Efficacy and safety of antifungal prophylaxis with oral itraconazole solution among patients receiving corticosteroids: who should be given prophylaxis? *J Infect Chemother* 2011;17:744-9.

Kaufman DA, Cuff AL, Wamstad JB, et al. Fluconazole prophylaxis in extremely low birth weight infants and neurodevelopmental outcomes and quality of life at 8 to 10 years of age. J Pediatr 2011;158:759-765.

Kim J, Sudbery P. *Candida albicans*, a major human fungal pathogen. J Microbiol 2011;49:171-177.

Kobayashi T, Kakeya H, Miyazaki T, et al. Synergistic antifungal effect of lactoferrin with azole antifungals against *Candida albicans* and a proposal for a new treatment method for invasive candidiasis. *Jpn J Infect Dis* 2011;64:292-296.

Lazzaro C. Economic evaluation of posaconazole in prophylaxis of invasive fungal infections in Italian neutropenic patients with acute myeloid leukaemia or myelodysplastic syndrome. *Infez Med* 2010;18:91-103.

Lyseng-Williamson KA. Posaconazole: a pharmacoeconomic review of its use in the prophylaxis of invasive fungal disease in immunocompromised hosts. *Pharmacoeconomics* 2011;29:251-68.

Mandal SM, Migliolo L, Franco OL, et al. Identification of an antifungal peptide from *Trapa natans* fruits with inhibitory effects on Candida tropicalis biofilm formation. *Peptides* 2011;32:1741-1747.

Méan M, Marchetti O, Calandra T. Bench-to-bedside review: Candida infections in the intensive care unit. *Crit Care.* 2008;12(1):204.

Ray A, Ray S, George AT, et al. Interventions for prevention and treatment of vulvovaginal candidiasis in women with HIV infection. *Cochrane Database Syst Rev* 2011;8:CD008739.

Reed BN, Caudle KE, Rogers PD. Fluconazole prophylaxis in high-risk neonates. *Ann Pharmacother* 2010;44:178-84.

Salavert M, Jarque I. Is micafungin useful in the prophylaxis of invasive fungal disease in hematological patients? *Enferm Infecc Microbiol Clin* 2011;29 Suppl 2:43-9.

San-Juan R, Aguado JM, Lumbreras C, et al. Universal prophylaxis with fluconazole for the prevention of early invasive fungal infection in low-risk liver transplant recipients. *Transplantation* 2011;92:346-50.

Scott LJ. Micafungin: a review of its use in the prophylaxis and treatment of invasive Candida infections. *Drugs.* 2012;72(16):2141-65.

Wang J, Zhan P, Zhou R, et al. Prophylaxis with itraconazole is more effective than prophylaxis with fluconazole in neutropenic patients with hematological malignancies: a meta-analysis of randomized-controlled trials. *Med Oncol* 2010;27:1082-8.

. Wilke M. Treatment and prophylaxis of invasive candidiasis with anidulafungin, caspofungin and micafungin and its impact on use and costs: review of the literature. *Eur J Med Res* 2011;16:180-6.

Wilkerson J, McPherson C, Donze A. Fluconazole to prevent systemic fungal infections in infants: reviewing the evidence. *Neonatal Netw* 2010;29:323-33.

Wong JH, Ng TB, Legowska A, et al. Antifungal action of human cathelicidin fragment (LL13-37) on *Candida albicans*. *Peptides* 2011;32:1996-2002.

In: Candida *albicans*: Symptoms, Causes and Treatment Options ISBN: 978-1-62808-882-3
Editors: Leon A. Dietrich and Tim S. Friedmann

Chapter XI

Candida albicans: New Aspects of Pathogenicity, Interaction to Antifungals, Biofilms and Preventive Anti-Candida Strategies – The Overview of Own Works

V. M. Lakhtin*[*], *M. V. Lakhtin, A. L. Bajrakova and S. S. Afanasiev

Department of Medical Biotechnology, G.N. Gabrichevsky Research Institute for Epidemiology and Microbiology, Moscow, Russia

Abstract

Own results, proposals, and conceptions published during last 5 years are summarized. *Candida albicans* and non-albicans Candida species isolated from urogenital tract of healthy people were compared in their interactions to antifungals (probiotic bacterial lectins [PBL] including bifidobacterial and lactobacillus lectins [BL, LL], phytolectins, antibiotics, lactobacilli) in suspensions and biofilms. Synergistic potential of antifungals against *Candida* species is presented. New prognostic and diagnostic features and criteria of *Candida albicans* strain pathogenicity according to both fungal behavior and fungal interaction to antimicrobials are proposed. Among *Candida* species strains tested, *C. albicans* strains reveal increased sensitivity to BL as well as to the block [ketokonazol, fluconazol] upon ranging antibiotic sensitivity.

Keywords: Candida albicans, non-albicans *Candida* species, microfungal body, lactobacilli, bifidobacteria, probiotics, synbiotics, antibiotics, probiotic lectins, pathogenicity, microbiocenoses, biotopes, mixed cultures, biofilms, prognostics, diagnostics

[*] E-mail: lakhtinv@yandex.ru.

Introduction [1-6]

Candida ssp. strains are initiator of different diseases in human organism when biotope balance between probiotic and relatively pathogenic microorganisms is altered. We studied *Candida* species strains isolated from intestinal and urogenital human biotopes (freshly isolated or museum strains from Collection of microorganisms of G.N. Gabrichevsky Research Institute for Epidemiology & Microbiology). The aim was to summarize own results, proposals and conceptions as minireview concerning additional and new *Candida albicans* aspects of fungal relative pathogenicity and including publications during last 5 years.

Behavior of *Candida albicans* Strains As Communicative Body [5, 7-11]

Microfungal body organization and functioning in stress conditions are useful for understanding its strategy and tactics, possible potential in biotope. It can be represented by associates, massives and/or biofilms. Its features include the presence of whole territory limited with borders of occupied landscape in center-peripheral and perimeter directions, own primitive center, central or internal (protected for higher survival, with increased multilayer distribution) and peripheral (around borders, with quick reactions to stress signals) regions connected each other by cell contacts, communicative signals between cells, layers or limited supracellular constructions (parts of body, pseudopodia, mosaic of independent islets as examples of pseudoorganogenesis). Coupled micro- or macrounit landscape "Empty Space - Hill" was observed as universal fungal unit reply (which can be summarized in center-peripheral and/or perimeter directions) to external (stress) or internal (according to development steps) signals of surrounding. Primitive library of visible image landscape collection of replies to stress signals including antifungals and physical factors decreased fungal territory in mosaic manner by conversion of primary one-center body into later multicenter one. Development and involution of body massive in conditions of prolonged stress allow monitoring main phenomena of fungal behavior, switching and other events of steps (sorbtion on and occupation of pore hydrophilic and hydrophobic sorbents, early biofilm forming, etc.). Among them it should be noted the primary growth of *C. albicans* massive before *Aspergillus niger* and *Penicillium ssp.*, as well as keeping resistance of *C. albicans* body regions without massive (due to region sensitivity to antifungals like probiotic bacterial lectins [PBL – carbohydrates/glycoconjugates-recognition polypeptides and their complexes]) to the presence of other fungal possible pathogens for prolonged time.

Sensor Character of Interactions between *Candida* and Antifungals [9, 12-14]

On the one hand, border (peripheral) regions of fungal body controlled territory can be used for sensor primary replies of fungi to stress signals including antifungals (PBL, phytolectins, antibiotics) and physical treatments. This is in contrast to central (internal) regions of increased body survival. Within functional group of *C. albicans* and *C. tropicalis* (the group with increased levels of expressed secreted hydrolases) highly sensitive (sensor) replies can be expected in case of specie *C. albicans*. Results indicate high synergistic anti-*Candida* potential of aforementioned antifungals of different types. On the other hand, *Lactobacillus* biotope populations can reveal highly sensitive behavior to the presence of *C. albicans* strains. *Lactobacillus* populations from the same biotope are able influence early *Candida* biofilms.

Potential of PBL in Study and Treatment of *Candida* [1-4]

PBL are new class of microbial pathogen biofilm destructors. They are of especial interest because of: their human origin, isolation from probiotic bacteria, standardization, biotope probiotic compartment- oriented and depended [lactobacilli as preferential regulating tool for urogenital tract, and bifidobacteria as preferential regulating tool for intestinal tract; combinations of lactobacillus and bifidobacterial PBL as universal for both biotopes]). PBL isolated from industrial probiotic *Lactobacillus* and bifidobacterial strains of human origin are perspective for large scale production to use as ingredients of antifungals. PBL can serve as key and important regulators of microbiocenoses in the directions "Microbes - Microbes" and "Microbes – Human organism". PBL are involved in regulation of biotope microbial populations. PBL serve as a key factor of biotope conversion into probiotic compartment. PBL can be used in screening probiotic and probiotic-like microbes, changed microbial populations and microbes with increased pathogenicity. As a result PBL are useful for evaluation of the biotope balance (healthy, intermediate, or non-healthy). Applications of PBL are multipotential and especially effective against eukaryotic pathogens like microfungi. PBL act as antipathogen cascade synergistic system (like bifidobacteria + lactobacilli) resulting in destruction of biofilms of relatively pathogenic microbiocenosis including genus *Candida* (biotope mixed relatively pathogenic compartment). Especially bifidobacterial acidic lectins possess high sensor features towards *C. albicans*. Compared to cell probiotics, PBL possess such advantages as reliable non-dangerous development of events in biotope, the possibility of simultaneous suppression of relatively pathogenic compartment and supporting probiotic compartment (also in cases when bifidobacteria and/or lactobacilli are currently absent in biotope). Synergistic actions between PBL and other antimicrobials (antibiotics, phytolectins, etc.) allow use of PBL in combinations. The latter can be important for decreasing final effective antibiotic doses upon treatments.

New Aspects of *Candida* Species and Strain Relative Pathogenicity

Within genus *Candida*, *Candida albicans* and non-albicans *Candida* species strains were compared. Additional evaluations of *Candida* species and strain relative pathogenicity (as factors of disease risk) were developed. Approaches included grouping (*C. albicans* and *C. tropicalis* as the same functional group which differs from *C. krusei and C. glabrata*; PBL as potential inactivators of important fungal hydrolases), relationship between *C. albicans* strain sensitivity to antibiotics [position of block "ketoconazol, fluconazol" decreased in a set *C. albicans C. tropicalis, C. krusei*; for local population of strain donors investigated], opposite coupled relationship as "Higher *Candida* specie virulence – Higher *Candida* specie sensitivity to PBL" (evolutionary developed protection reply of probiotic microorganisms [especially for bifidobacteria] against activated metabolic activities of fungi in biotope). Additional approaches included fungal body behavior monitoring (also in the presence of antimicrobials) when visible action of mosaic attack of antifungals (including PBL) in respect of *C. albicans* strains can be compared in inhibition of growth (strain resistance as factor of risk), limited or complete destruction (strain resistance as factor of risk), the presence of wave type distribution of massive changing (the presence as factor of risk), survival upon prolonged stress (factor of risk), etc. Aforementioned approaches developed served as the basis for proposals on potential preventive antifungal strategies (see below). It seems, additional landscape criteria of increased relative pathogenicity of *C. albicans* strain can be: a) keeping fungal body territory as mostly resistant to the presence of PBL – imitators of probiotics; b) increased fungal resistance to combinations of PBL (BL and LL; acidic and/or cationic PBL), PBL and some antibiotics (some azoles, nystatin, amphotericin B) or lectins-containing some phytopreparations of medical significance; c) strain capability to produce own associates-dissolving activity (as step needed for early growth); d) resistance to the presence of lactobacilli from the same biotope in reaction of early mixed biofilm forming (when lactobacilli not influence fungal biofilm forming).

Antifungal Strategies [5, 7-9, 15-26]

Results indicate the following number of potential preventive anti-*Candida* strategies:

- The main biotopes for anti-*Candida* treatments can be represented by rectal (preferential action of bifidobacteria and PBL) and urogenital (preferential action of lactobacilli and PBL) tracts. PBL as imitators of probiotics have advantages of using as non-cellular system forms (formulas) especially in cases of dysbiotic absence of bifidobacteria and/or lactobacilli in biotopes.
- The use of fungal sensor landscape regions for quick antifungal attack (biochemical or/and physical) to reach quick result of significant decreasing or limitation of fungal body.
- The use of mosaic multiple point/spot type distribution of PBL all over fungal body (acidic or cationic PBL in peripheral or internal regions, respectively). Other synergistic action of LL and BL (characterized with different sets of glycoconjugate targets; possessing potential of recognizing simple glycoantigens) may be used against different *Candida* populations of the fungal body (directly or in delivery cofunctioning constructions). As a result communicative death of the fungal body can be reached.

- PBL in combinations with other antifungal types: a) antibiotics to decrease work antibiotic doses and for alternative treatments against multidrug-resistant fungal strains; b) phytolectins-containing phytopreparations to extend mechanisms of antifungal actions of combinations.
- Combinations of antifungals with physical factors for treatments.
- Increasing antifungal potential by the use of system of PBL-glycoconjugates (pseudopolysaccharides of mucin type) complexes.
- Different probiotic bacteria (for example, *Lactobacillus*) populations (with increased biofilm decstructing activities or *Candida* cell associated activity) may be used against different *Candida* populations (with increased biofilm forming activities or *Candida* cell producing hydrolase activities).
- Consideration of local (biotope type in organism, geographic position) features of populations of peoples (extending probiotic compartment in antifungal combinative compositions by introducing adequate key probiotic bacterial strains and/or combinations of PBL into sym/synbiotic mixtures).
- Personalized (individual) approaches for patient treatments (probiotic part of antifungal sym/synbiotic composition may include imitation of intrinsic probiotic-like compartment [as model combinations of probiotic-like strains isolated from uroginital or intestinal biotope] of individual patient concrete biotope). In this respect possible intrinsic extended biotope sym/synbiotic consortia (probiotic bacteria + PBL) analysis is of especial usefulness for choice and development of perspective strategy in natural adaptation and stabilization of the probiotic biotope microbial individual compartment.

Conclusion [3, 26]

It seems, observed interactions *of Candida* species strains and antifungals may allow prediction of possible effective anti-*Candida* synergistic (in space and time) combinations, cascade regimes and other special conditions (multiple mosaic point attack within fungal body) of using antifungals against fungal associates, massives or biofilms. The data obtained indicate potential of new combinations of anti-*Candida* coctails including PBL as imitators of probiotics and ingredients of synbiotics. The use of biotope pro/symbiotic [delivered] or pro/synbiotic-like [intrinsic] microbial consortia (in cases of virtual biotope of people population or individual one) is perspective for antifungal strategies and tactics (for example, against *C. albicans*) as well as for population and individual medicine. The data obtained are also of interest for medical nutrition in development of new pro/symbiotic-like products when natural multifunctional antimicrobial (including antifungal) combinations can be rationally used.

References

[1] Lakhtin MV, Aleshkin VA, Lakhtin VM, Nesvizhsky YV, Afanasiev SS, et al. (2010) [The Role of Lectins from Probiotic Microorganisms in Sustaining the Macroorganism (in Russian)]. *Vestnik Rossiiskoy Academii Meditsinskih Nauk* (Moskva) [*Vestnik of Russian Academy of Medical Sciences* (Moscow)] 2: 3-8. ISSN 0869-6047.

[2] Lakhtin M, Aleshkin V, Lakhtin V, Afanasiev S, Pozhalostina L, Pospelova V (2010) Probiotic Lactobacillus and Bifidobacterial Lectins against *Candida albicans* and *Staphylococcus aureus* clinical Strains: New Class of Pathogen Biofilm Destructors. *Probiotics & Antimicrobial Proteins* 2: 186-196. DOI: 10.1007/s12602-010-9046-3.

[3] Lakhtin M., Lakhtin V., Aleshkin A., Bajrakova A., Afanasiev S., Aleshkin V. (2012) Lectin Systems imitating Probiotics: Potential for Biotechnology and medical Microbiology. In: *"Probiotics 2012"*, Edited by E.C. Rigobelo, http://dx.doi.org/10/5772/3444. InTech. P. 417–432. ISBN 978-953-51-0776-7.

[4] Lakhtin MV, Bajrakova AL, Lakhtin VM, Afanasiev SS, Aleshkin VA (2012) [Lectins of Probiotics – New Class of Signal Molecules of Quorum sensing (in Russian)]. *Klinitcheskaya laboratornaya diagnostika* (Moskva) [*Clinical Laboratory Diagnostics* (Moscow)] No 9: 82-83. ISSN 0869-2084.

[5] Lakhtin VM, Lakhtin MV, Afanasiev SS (2012) [The Fight for Space and Resources between probiotic and relatively pathogenic Compartments in potential Biotope: Lectin Type Imitators of Probiotics against eukaryotic Pathogens – Importance for Biotechnology (in Russian)]. In: *Proceedings of the VIII International Conference "Key questions in Modern Science"* (April 17 – 25, Sofia, Bulgaria). Sofia, Vol. 28: 28 – 33. [*Материали за 8-а международна научна практична конференция, «Ключови въпроси в съвременната наука»*, - 2012. 28: 28 – 33. Биологии. Селско стопанство. София. «Бял ГРАД-БГ» ООД]. ISBN 978-966-8736-05-6.

[6] Lakhtin VM, Lakhtin MV, Agapova YV, Belikova YV, Kulakova YV, Afanasiev SS, Alehkin VA (2012) Advantadges of the Probiotic "Acilact" compared to Ingredient Strains using algorithmic Ranges of Qualities. In: *Proceedings of the VIII International Conference "Scientific Space of Europe - 2012"* (April 7-15, Przemyśl. Poland). Przemyśl, Nauka i studia. Vol. 32: 50 – 57. *Materiały VIII Międzynarodowej naukowi-praktycznej konferencji «Naukowa przestrzeń Europy - 2012»* Vol. 32. – P. 50-57. Nauk biologicznych: Przemyśl. Nauka i studia. ISBN 978-966-8736-05-6.

[7] Lakhtin MV, Lakhtin VM, Aleshkin VA, Afanasiev SS, et al. (2009) Antifungal Potential of Probiotic bacterial Lectin Preparations and Phytopreparations: Types, Mechanisms and Factors of Actions against Human Pathogenic Microfungi. *Practical Phytotherapy* No 4: 17-25.

[8] Lakhtin MV, Lakhtin VM, Aleshkin VA, Afanasiev SS, Korsun VF (2010) [Phyto- and Probiotic Lectins – Synergistic Antipathogens (in Russian)]. *Praktitcheskaya fitoterapiya* (Moskva) [*Practical Phytotherapy* (Moscow)] No 1: 5-11. ISBN5-88010-096-0.

[9] Lakhtin MV, Lakhtin VM, Aleshkin VA, Bajrakova AL, Afanasiev SS, Korsun VF (2011) [Phyto- and Probiotic-Analog Therapy of microfungal Infections: Theory and Practice Potential in Development (in Russian)]. *ARS Medica* No 15: 183-187. ISSN 2220-5497.

[10] Lakhtin MV, Lakhtin VM, Aleshkin AV, Bajrakova AL, Afanasiev SS, Aleshkin VA, Korsun VF (2012) [Probiotic Lectins – Ingredients of Biopreparations, Bioadditives and Drug Forms (in Russian)]. *Praktitcheskaya fitoterapiya* (Moskva) *[Practical Phytotherapy* (Moscow)] No 1: 4-9. ISBN5-88010-096-0.

[11] Lakhtin MV, Afanasyev SS, Lakhtin VM, Bajrakova AL, Aleshkin AV, Korsun VF (2013) [Probiotic Lectins of different Origin in combinative Therapy (in Russian)]. *Electronic Science & Education Vestnik "Health in XXI Century"* (Moscow). 15; No 3: 14-17. ISSN 2226-7417. URL: http://e-pubmed.org/isu15-3.html.

[12] Lakhtin MV, Bajrakova AL, Lakhtin VM, Afanasiev SS, Aleshkin VA (2012) [*Lactobacillus* Populations as Biotope Sensor sensitive to the Presence of Lectins of Human Probiotic Bacteria (in Russian)]. *Klinitcheskaya laboratornaya diagnostika* (Moskva) [*Clinical Laboratory Diagnostics* (Moscow)] No 9: 83. ISSN 0869-2084.

[13] Lakhtin VM, Bajrakova AL, Lakhtin MV, Belikova YV, Afanasiev SS, Aleshkin VA (2012) [Regulating Properties of the Human Probiotic bacterial Consortium Lectins: Screening, Modulation and Selection of Normoflora of *Lactobacillus* populations from the same Biotope (in Russian)]. In: *Proceedings of the VIII International Conference "Days of Science"*. Prague, Vol. 74: 38 – 44. [*Materiály VIII mezinárodní vědecko - praktická conference «Dny vědy - 2012»*. - Díl 74: 38 – 44. Biologické vědy: Praha. Publishing House «Education and Science» s.r.o.]. ISBN 978-966-8736-05-6.

[14] Lakhtin VM, Bajrakova AL, Lakhtin MV, Afanasiev SS. (2013) [Modulation of early Biofilms by Human microbial Consortia: Conception of extended Biotope Probiotic Compartment, prognostic Patterns (in Russian)]. In: *Proceedings of the VI Conference "Moderrn Technologies and Methods of Diagnostics of Different Groups of Diseases, Laboratory Analysis"* (23-24 May 2013, Moscow). Book of Abstracts: 21-22.

[15] Lakhtin VM, Dykhal YI, Lakhtin MV, et al. BA (2009) New Lectin Systems in cultural Fluids of Probiotic Strains of Lactobacilli and Bifidobacteria capable to discriminate Glycoantigens containing GalNAc. *Gastroenterologia Sankt-Peterburga* [*Gastroenterology of Sankt-Petersburg*] No 4: A14-A15. ISSN 1727-7906.

[16] Lakhtin V, Aleshkin V, Lakhtin M, Afanasiev S (2009) Glycoconjugates in Discrimination of Glycoconjugate Recognition Systems of Probiotic Microorganisms. New Potential Keys for Strains and Glycometabolome typing. *Glycoconjugate Journal.* 26: 876.

[17] Lakhtin VM, Aleshkin VA, Bajrakova AL, Lakhtin MV, Afanasiev SS, et al. (2010) Screening clinical Strains of *Candida tropicalis, C. krusei, C. glabrata* and *C. albicans* using Antibiotics and Lectins of Human Probiotic Bacteria (in Russian)]. *Klinitcheskaya laboratornaya diagnostika* (Moskva) [*Clinical Laboratory Diagnostics* (Moscow)] No 9: 37. ISSN 0869-2084.

[18] Lakhtin MV, Lakhtin VM, Cherepanova YV, Pospelova VV, Afanasiev SS, Aleshkin VA (2011) Ranging Qualities of industrial Ingredient Probiotic Strains of Human Bifidobacteria and Lactobacilli to predict New Probiotic Formulas. In: *Proceedings of International Conference "Modern Achievements of Biotechnology"* (June 21-23, 2011, Stavropol, Russia). Part 2. Division "Bioadditives". Moscow: NOU "Education Scientific Technical Center of Milk Industry", 49 – 51.

[19] Lakhtin MV, Bajrakova AL, Lakhtin VM, Aleshkin AV, Afanasiev SS, Aleshkin VA (2011) [Microbiocenosis Model "Pathogen – Probiotic Lectins" for monitoring Primate Biotope Dysbioses (in Russian)]. *Proceedings of the 2nd International Scientific*

Conference "Fundamental and Applied Aspects of Medical Primatology" (August 8-10, 2011, Sochi, Russia). Vol. 1. Sochi: 88-92.

[20] Lakhtin MV, Bajrakova AL, Lakhtin VM, Afanasiev SS, Aleshkin VA, et al. (2011) [Probiotic Lectins of Human in Protection against Dysbioses in different Human Biotopes (in Russian)]. *Praktitcheskaya fitoterapiya* (Moskva) [*Practical Phytotherapy* (Moscow)] No 1: 4-13. ISBN5-88010-096-0.

[21] Lakhtin MV, Aleshkin VA, Lakhtin VM, Galimzyanov HM, Afanasiev SS, Karaulov AV, Nesvijskyi YV, Bajrakova AL, et al. (2011) Behavior of Pathogenic Fungi of Genus *Candida* in the Presence of Probiotic Lectins. *Astrakhan Medical Journal* 6(2):73-76. ISSN 1992-6499.

[22] Lakhtin MV, Aleshkin VA, Lakhtin VM Afanasiev SS, Karaulov AV, Galimzyanov HM, Nesvijskyi YV, Bajrakova AL, et al. (2011) Behavior of *Candida tropicalis* and *Candida krusei* in the Presence of Probiotic Lectins. *Astrakhan Medical Journal* 6(3): 97-101. ISSN 1992-6499.

[23] Lakhtin MV, Kozlov LV, Lakhtin VM, Aleshkin VA, Afanasiev SS, et al. (2012) [Protection of Human potential Antibodies from *Candida* cclinical Strain Secret Proteolysis in the Presence of Lectins of Human Probiotic Bacteria (in Russian)]. *Astrakhan Medical Journal* 7(1): 63–68. ISSN 1992-6499.

[24] Lakhtin M, Lakhtin V, Bajrakova A, Aleshkin A, Afanasiev S, Aleshkin V (2012) Interaction of Probiotic Bacterial Lectins to *Candida* Species. In: Proceedings of the VIII International Conference "*Sciences and Technology: Step in Future*" (Feb. 27 – March 5, Prague, Chechia). – Vol. 29: 34 - 41. Materiály VIII mezinárodní vědecko - praktická conference «Věda a technologie: krok do budoucnosti - 2012». - Díl 29: 34 – 41. Biologické vědy: Praha. Publishing House «Education and Science». ISBN 978-966-8736-05-6.

[25] Lakhtin MV, Karaulov AV, Lakhtin VM, Aleshkin VA, Afanasiev SS, et al. (2012) [*Lectin – Glycoconjugate Systems in Human* Organism (in Russian)]. Immunopathology, Allergology, Infectology (Moscow) No 1: 27-36. ISSN 0236-297X.

[26] Lakhtin MV, Aleshkin VA, Lakhtin VM, Nesvizhsky YV, Afanasiev SS, et al. (2012) [Prospects of Lectins of Probiotics in Chemotherapy (in Russian)]. In: *Proceedings of the VIII International Conference "Days of Science"* (March 27 – April 5, Prague, Chechia). Prague, Publishing House «Education and Science» s.r.o. Vol. 74: 6 – 10. Materiály VIII mezinárodní vědecko - praktická conference «Dny vědy - 2012». - Díl 74: 6 – 10. Biologické vědy: Praha. Publishing House «Education and Science» s.r.o. ISBN 978-966-8736-05-6.

In: Candida *albicans*: Symptoms, Causes and Treatment Options ISBN: 978-1-62808-882-3
Editors: Leon A. Dietrich and Tim S. Friedmann

Chapter XII

Vaginal Candidiasis and its Risk Factors among Women Attending a Nigerian Teaching Hospital

S. I. Nwadioha[1,*], E .O. P. Nwokedi[2], J. Egesie[2] and H. Enejuo[3]
[1]Department of Medical Microbiology&Parasitology, College of Health Sciences, Benue State University,Makurdi.Nigeria
[2]Department of Haematology, Jos University Teaching Hospital, Jos. Nigeria
[3]Department of Microbiology&Parasitology , Aminu Kano Teaching Hospital, Kano Nigeria
Study Site: Aminu Kano Teaching Hospital, Kano Nigeria

Abstract

Aims and Objectives: The study was set to detect *Candida* species in female genital discharge and validate the associated risk factors by laboratory means.

Materials and Methods: A prospective study of female genital swabs collected from women with abnormal vaginal discharge (test group) and a control group who were attending gynecology, family planning, antenatal care or HIV/STI clinics of Aminu Kano Teaching Hospital, Kano Nigeria and analysed for microscopy and culture in microbiology laboratory from December 2008 to December 2009. Data on epidemiologic indices were collected from the patients, using structured interviewer- administered questionnaires.

Results: Candida species were detected in the test group in 60% (n=600/1000) cases of infective vaginal discharge while 12% (120/1000) in the control group . The isolation rate of *Candida albicans* was 69% more than the non- albicans. Distribution of vaginal candidiasis in the test group, was prevalent in young adults age group of 21 to 30 years

* Correspondence to: S.I. Nwadioha, Department of Medical Microbiology, & Parasitology, College of Health Sciences, Benue State University,Makurdi.Nigeria. Email: samnwa2000@yahoo.com
Phone: +234- 08056838967

with 50% (n=300/600), in patients with pregnancy 38% (n=225/600) and patients with chronically debilitating illnesses 26% (n=157/600).

Conclusion: The result shows that vaginal candidiasis is quite common and *Candida albicans* is the most prevalent species. We therefore recommend early diagnosis and prompt treatment of vaginal candidiasis in all women clinics especially among the patients with chronic debilitating illness, pregnancy and young adults in order to avert the complications of vaginal candidiasis and reduce HIV transmission.

Keywords: Vaginal candidiasis, risk factors, microscopy, culture

Introduction

Vaginal Candidiasis is a common type of vaginitis, a gynecologic disorder that manifests with an odorless curdy white discharge ("cottage cheese") in the female lower reproductive tracts with pruritus, irritation, dysuria or dyspareunia [1]. It is a common complaint among women of different age groups in any society whether or not they are sexually active. Some studies have shown high preponderance of vaginal candidiasis in infective vaginal discharge with 42 to 52.5% isolation rate of *candida* species [1, 2].

Risk factors for vaginal candidiasis are factors that do not seem to be a direct cause of the disease, but seem to be associated in some way. Having the risk factor makes the chances of the condition higher but does not always lead to vaginal candidiasis. Also, the absence of any risk factors or having a protective factor does not necessarily guard one against vaginal candidiasis [3]. Some of the risk factors include pregnancy, poorly controlled diabetes, oral contraceptive, antibiotics, immune suppression in chronic debilitating illness like HIV, tuberculosis and cancer, douches, perfumed feminine hygiene sprays, topical antimicrobial agents, tight clothing, tight under- wears, thyroid disorders and corticosteroid [3].

Vaginal candidiasis is caused by the fungus *Candida albicans* in approximately 85% of cases, while other species such as *C. glabrata, C. krusei, C. tropicalis* and *C. stellatoidea* rarely cause vaginitis [4]. *Candida* species are usually of endogenous origin and may be transmitted by sexual partners. Changes in the vaginal environment are usually necessary before the organism can induce pathological effects.

Although vaginal candidiasis is both treatable and mild, when left untreated, is a possible risk for acquisition of HIV/AIDS as well as other complications [5]. Other complications include pelvic inflammatory disease, infertility, ectopic pregnancy, pelvic abscess, menstrual disorders, spontaneous abortion and premature birth. It is now well established that the presence of infective vaginal discharge greatly facilitates transmission and acquisition of HIV between sexual partners [6].

Therefore, there is a need for early diagnosis and prompt treatment of this common condition especially among the risk groups, in order to avert the complications and reduce the transmission of HIV. Laboratory support is necessary for a differential diagnosis or to confirm the clinical diagnosis of vaginal candidiasis. The purpose of this study was to investigate vaginal candidiasis among female patients attending Aminu Kano Teaching Hospital Kano, northwestern Nigeria, in order to achieve an effective medical management of this condition.

Materials and Methods

This descriptive study was carried out from December 2008 to December 2009 in Aminu Kano Teaching Hospital Kano, Nigeria. Approval of the study protocol was obtained from the ethics committee of the hospital.

Consent of the patients was sought and received. Genital swabs were collected from patients with abnormal vaginal discharge who presented in gynecology clinics, family planning clinics, antenatal clinics, HIV/STIs clinics. Also, genital swabs were collected from similar population who attended same clinics but did not have abnormal vaginal discharge, to serve as control. Data were collected from the patients using a structured interviewer-administered questionnaire. Endo-cervical and high- vaginal samples were collected from the patients for laboratory analysis. *Specimen collection:* The patient lied on examining table in supine position with the thighs extended. The procedure was carried out in a sterile condition with sterile hand gloves. With the patient in the lithotomy position, any copious discharge running out into the perineum was cleaned off, the labia were spread with a gloved hand, and a sterile vaginal speculum moistened with warm water was gently inserted; the vaginal walls and cervix were examined. High vaginal swab was collected from the posterior and lateral fornices of the vagina with a sterile cotton swab stick. A second cotton swab stick was used to collect specimen from the endocervical canal. After the speculum was gently withdrawn and patient was cleaned up. A characteristic fishy odor was intensified by adding a drop of 10% potassium hydroxide (KOH) to the vaginal fluid on the examination speculum (WHIFF Test for Bacterial vaginosis).

Laboratory Procedures

The genital swabs were immediately sent to the genital bench of Medical Microbiology and Parasitology laboratory, where they were processed according to standard procedures [4]. Infection with *Candida* species was diagnosed by microscopy of a saline mount, Gram-stained smear of material from the vagina and colonial growth on Sabouraud's Dextrose agar. *Microscopy*: Saline Mount.

A saline mount of the vaginal discharge specimen was covered with a cover- slip, and examined microscopically at ×40 objective, not only to detect yeast cells, but to exclude the presence of trichomonads and clue cells. Yeasts are round ovoid cells, 4µm in diameter, showing typical budding (blastoconidia). Yeasts can easily be recognized on a Gram stained smear as Gram- positive cells. Bacterial vaginosis was further diagnosed by examining ten fields of high power (x40) objective for clue cells (epithelial cells heavily coated bacteria sufficient to obscure the cell borders) for Bacteria vaginosis. *Trichomonas vaginalis* was diagnosed by microscopy of a saline mount for the actively motile, spear shaped flagellates. Gram-stained smear. Vaginal smears were Gram-stained. (a) Microscopic evaluation of Gram –stained smear at high power (x40) objective revealed clue cells, usually representing at least 20 percent of vaginal epithelial cells in BV. (b) At oil immersion power (x100) objective, Gram- stain scores of 0 -10 were assigned on basis of standardized criteria (Nugent); with 0 representing *Lactobacilli* (large Gram-positive rods) predominant vaginal flora while at the extreme 10 representing flora predominated by *Gardnerella, Bacteroides* and *Mobilincus* organisms (small Gram-negative or variable or curved rods). Scores of 0 – 3 were considered normal, 4 -6 borderline for BV and 7 -10 diagnostic of BV. A score ≥4 was used to define abnormal vaginal flora.

Culture: Antibiotic treated selective Sabouraud dextrose agar (SDA) was used as a growth medium for the isolation of *Candida* species. After inoculation of the clinical specimen, plates were incubated at 36°C for 2 days. Colonies of yeast cells are opaque white to creamy. Identification: A simple test for the presumptive identification of *C. albicans* is the germ tube test. A colony was emulsified in 0.5ml – 1ml of sterile serum and incubated at 35 - 37°C for 4 hours. *C. albicans* form germ tubes, short lateral hyphal filaments without any constrictions. It was examined every half hour for formation of germ tubes.

Some rare *C. albicans* do not grow germ tubes.

In the past, it has been emphasized that *C. stellatoidea* also produces germ tube, and distinction between *C. albicans* should be made. Now, *C. stellatoidea* is no longer a valid species and has been combined with *C. albicans* [4]. The germ tube is specific for the identification of *C. albicans*, with the exception of an occasional isolate of *C. tropicalis* that may rarely produce germ tube.

Table 1. *Candida* species detected in the Test group in Aminu Kano Teaching Hospital Nigeria, December 2008 to December 2009

No. of genital swabs	Types of Microbes	No. of Microbes	%
1000	*Candida albicans*	412	41
1000	Non albicans *spp.*	188	19
1000	Other microbes (* *T. vag.*, *N. gonorr.*and agents of BV including *G. vag.*)	180	18
1000	Non pathogens	40	4

*T. vag. =Trichomonas vaginalis, BV= Bacterial vaginosis, G. vag.=Gardenerella vaginalis, N. gonorr=Neisseria gonorrhoeae, Spp.=species.

**40 samples had multiple isolates.

Table 2. *Candida* species detected in the Control group in Aminu Kano Teaching Hospital Nigeria, December 2008 to December 2009

No. of genital swabs	Types of Microbes	No. of Microbes	%
1000	*Candida albicans*	100	10
1000	Non albicans spp.	20	2
1000	Other microbes (* *T. vag.*, *N. gonorr.*and agents of BV including *G. vag.*)	0	0
1000	Non pathogens	300	30

*T. vag. =Trichomonas vaginalis, BV= Bacterial vaginosis, G. vag.=Gardenerella vaginalis, N. gonorr=Neisseria gonorrhoeae, Spp.=species.

Table 3. Candida species detected in the test group and the control group

Sample groups	Genital swabs	*Candida* species (*C. albicans* and Non albicans) detected	%
Test group	1000	600(412+188)	60
Control group	1000	120(100+20)	12

$X^2 = 45.91$ df=1 P = 0.00002.

Table 4. Distribution of vaginal candidiasis in relation to pregnancy, contraceptives, broad spectrum antibiotics and chronic debilitating illness among study population

Age in years	Vaginal Candid-iasis	Pregnant women	Contraceptives	Broad spectrum antibiotics	Chronically debilitating illness	Undete-rmined factors
0-10	5	-	-	-	1	4
11-20	100	15	20	10	22	33
21-30	300	150	80	24	46	
31-40	100	60	10	15	15	
41-50	70	-	-	17	53	
51-60	25	-	-	5	20	
Total	600	225(38%)	110(18%)	71(12%)	157(26%)	37(6%)

A complete identification of *Candida* species was done by means of "sugar assimilation test" (auxanogram) by Wickerham-Burton method. The yeast was grown on a basal carbohydrate-free medium supplemented with essential vitamins and the test sugar. Each of the five test sugars, namely; glucose (positive control), sucrose, trehalose, lactose and raffinose was dispensed into each plate. Plates were incubated at 30°C for 48 hours. Growth produces an opacity in the medium and indicates the ability of the isolates to assimilate a sugar. *C. albicans* assimilate glucose, sucrose and trehalose only; *C. stellatoidea* assimilates glucose and trehalose only; *C. tropicalis* assimilates glucose, sucrose and trehalose only; *C. krusei* assimilates glucose only; *C. paratropicalis* assimilates glucose, sucrose,lactose and raffinose only; *C. parapsilosis* assimilates glucose, sucrose and trehalose only; *C. guilliermondi* assimilates glucose, sucrose, trehalose and raffinose.

Cervical specimens were Gram –stained and cultures were inoculated on plates of Chocolates and Thayer-Martin (Oxoid) media and incubated at 37° C in a moisturized candle extinction jar for 24 to 72 hours. *Neisseria gonorrhoeae* was identified by typical colonial morphology, reactions to Gram-stain, positive Oxidase test, and sugar fermentation. The antibiotic sensitivity of isolates was tested by the agar diffusion method on chocolate agar plates using oxoid multidiscs with standard antibiotic concentrations. The samples collection, transportation and processing including microscopy, culture and biochemical tests were carried out according to recommended standard [4]

The results were analysed using SPSS 11.0 statistical software; chi-square(x^2) was used to compare association between proportions and p-values<0.05 were considered significant at 95.0% confidence level.

Discussion

Vaginal candidiasis was a leading cause of infective vaginal discharge in the study with 60% (n=600/1000) prevalent rate in the test group. The prevalence of vaginal candidiasis in the control group was 12% (n=120/1000). The finding showed a steady rise of 52.5% [2] to 60% in prevalence of vaginal candidiasis in high vaginal swabs collected from infective vaginal discharges from 2003 to 2009 in Aminu Kano Teaching Hospital, Kano. The steady rise in vaginal candidiasis may be attributed to HIV/AIDS and other debilitating illnesses and behavioral changes in the changing society. *Candida* is a normal flora, but the overgrowth becomes pathogenic. Predominance of candidiasis in the study was in the young adult age group (21 -30 years). The age group of 21 -30 is the most sexually active group with highest risk of pregnancies, indulgence in family planning pills and immunosuppression due to HIV/AIDS [2]. The inflammation of the vagina, as in any inflammatory STI, increases the risk of acquisition of HIV [3]

Candida albicans isolated in the test group was 69% (n=412/600) of the total *Candida* species while n*on albicans* contributed 31% (n=188/600). The predominance of *C. albicans* in the result was in keeping with another study [4], which reported that vaginal candidiasis is created by the fungus *Candida albicans* in approximately 85% of cases, with non- albicans being responsible for the remaining 15%. An explanation for the predominance of *C. albicans* in the study may be that these species are more predominant than other C*andida* species in the environment and hence more in human body. More importantly, is their favorable survival ability in a depressed human immune system.

Pregnant mothers constituted 38% of the total case of vaginal candidiasis in the study. Some other studies have implicated pregnancy as an important risk factor for vaginitis [5, 6, 7]. The relationship between pregnancy and vaginal candidiasis may be due to increase in hormonal influences and alteration in vaginal PH [6, 5]. The rate of vaginal candidiasis among patients on contraceptives was 18%. The study included patients on oral or injects, implants or IUCD. Hormonal therapy leads to an inter-play between hormonal influences and alteration in vaginal PH [7, 5]. The normal mature vagina has a PH of 4.0.

Patients of chronically debilitating illnesses recorded 26% risk in the study. Systemic condition such as uncontrolled diabetic mellitus, HIV/AIDS, organ transplants, cancer and immunosuppressant drugs can increase the woman's chances of developing vulvovaginal candiasis [8, 3]. Depressed cell mediated immunity and dysfunction of neutrophils and monocytes provide a favorable condition for growth of *Candida* species such as in HIV/AIDS and diabetes mellitus respectively [9, 5, 6, 3].

The rate of vaginal candiasis in patients on a long term broad spectrum antibiotics in the study was 12%. Antibiotics and vaginal douching suppress normal bacterial flora and allow *Candida* organisms to proliferate. Of interest is that sulfonamide decrease neutrophil intracellular killing of C*andida* organisms and tetracyclines and amino glycosides have been shown to decrease neutrophil phagocytosis [10, 8, 3].

Early diagnosis and prompt treatment of vaginal candidiasis especially among the chronically debilitated ill patients, pregnant mothers, long term broad spectrum antibiotics users and young female adults must be implemented in order to avert the complications and reduce HIV transmission.

Conclusion

The result shows that *Candida* species is still a leading cause of vaginitis. Therefore, a high index of suspicion of candidiasis should be placed on the risk groups in a bid to control HIV acquisition and transmission.

References

[1] Nwadioha SI, Egah DZ, Nwokedi EOP, Odimayo MS. A study of female genital swabs in primary health care centres in Jos, Nigeria. *J. Med. & Pharm. Sci.*, 2009;5(1):95-98.

[2] Nwokedi EE, Anyiam NN. A study of high vaginal swabs in Kano. Teaching Hospital. A preliminary report *J. Highland. Med. Res.*, 2003; 1:57-61.

[3] John EE. Mycosis. In: Mandell, Bennett & Dollin .Editors. Textbook of Principles and Practice of Infectious Diseases. 5th Ed. New York: Churchill Livingstone, 2000. Pp.2291.

[4] Betty A, Forbes, Daniel FS, Alice SW. Editors. Genital Infections. In: laboratory manual of Bailey & Scotts diagnostic microbiology. 12th Ed. *Mosby Elsevier publication,* 2007. Pp. 753-872.

[5] Nwadioha SI, Egah DZ, Banwat EB, Alao OO. Microbial agents of abnormal vaginal discharge in pregnant mothers attending PHC clinics of Jos Nigeria. *J. Clin. Med. & Res.,* 2009;2:007-011. At http//www.academicjournals.org/JCMR.

[6] Federal Ministry of Health, Department of Public Health, National AIDS/STI Control Programme. Technical report 2010: National HIV/Syphilis sero-prevalence sentinel survey among pregnant women attending antenatal clinics in Nigeria. *Abuja;* 2010: 1-11.

[7] Omole – Ohonsi A, Mohammed Z, Ihesiulor U. Vaginal discharge in Pregnancy in Kano, Northern Nigeria. *Nig. Med. Pract.,* 2006; 50:68 -71.

[8] Jombo GTA, Opajobi SO, Egah DZ, Banwat EB, Denen Akaa P.. Symptomatic vulvovaginal candidiasis and genital colonization by candida species in Nigeria. *J Pub Hlth & Epidem,* 2010; 2(6):147-151. At http//www.academicjournals.org/JPHE.

[9] Akerele J. Abdul P. Okonufua F. Prevalence of asymptomatic genital infection among pregnant women in Benin city . Nigeria. *Afri. J. Reprod. Hlth.,* 2002; 6(3): 93-97.

[10] Anderson MR, Klink K, Cohrsen A. Evaluation of vaginal complaints. *JAMA,* 2000; 291: 1368.

Index

D

E

F

G

H

I

J

K

L

M

N

O

P

T

U

V

W

X

Y

Z